Make a Difference...A Practical Approach to Dementia Care

By

Deborah A. Bastedo, MA, NCC, LLPC, tLLP

and

Angela Willis, RN, BSN, MS, NHA

(doctoral candidate)

ISBN: 0-7596-8317-4

This book is printed on acid free paper.

First Edition Published in 1998 by Bastedo, MRS, Inc., 1069 Pelham Blvd., Waterford, MI 48328

Editor: Randall L. Bastedo
Editor for Understanding: Ruth Savakinas
Portrait of David Terry and Cover Design by John R. Bastedo, BAA; **Graphic Artist**

Clip Art © IXLA, LTD 1997-1998

The Pastoral Ministry section may be used with author acknowledgment.

Prologue

There is a lot more to a person and their physical, emotional and spiritual health than the questions asked during medical assessment of a person who has dementia would imply. We rely on the keen eyesight and good judgment of daily caregivers to identify areas of need. Every time a caregiver enters a room, he or she is noticing what this person is like. Of all the hard work and wonderful things which may be done, sometimes changes in condition occur which are not recognized as changes when a resident has dementia; that is, he or she has a new problem. But this current problem is not thought to be dementia because new symptoms are often seen as behavior problems rather than something new. We need to look for other possible reasons why this person is acting the way he or she is acting. Physicians often treat new problems as psychosis or mental illness behavior rather than potential indicators of a medical problem. An example would be hitting the caregiver, which may be an indicator of pain caused by the movement of joints during dressing rather than a symptom of psychosis or mental illness.

Please do not feel bad about this; many caregivers are just now beginning to identify the language of confusion.

Most caregivers I have had the pleasure to work with are dedicated and hardworking, and respond to the person's needs. However, They do not always understand what a confused person's behavior is communicating to them. Just as each nation has its own language with different countries having different dialects, each demented person has his or her own adaptation of the dialect. In a way, it's like a Sherlock Holmes novel; caregivers need to put together the clues to attempt to determine what this person is really trying to tell them with his or her behavior. My father taught me to understand the language of Alzheimer's in his dialect. I have been able to successfully help with behavior management by following the clues each person gives to prevent the cause of inappropriate behavior. Rather than dealing with an angry, hitting, confused person. The purpose of this book is to provide the reader with IDEAS. It is not written by a medical expert. It is not written as an authoritative guide but rather a collection of memories and a collection of tried approaches which helped in caring for my confused father as well as other confused people.

Table Of Contents

Chapter 1   In The Beginning 1

Chapter 2   What Is Dementia? 3

Chapter 3   Factors To Rule Out Prior To Being Certain It Is Dementia (Sometimes Referred To As Mental Status Change.) 6

Is It Dementia Or Is It Delirium? 9

Is It Dementia Or Is It Depression? 10

Chapter 4   Why Do They Do The Things They Do? 12

Chapter 5   Once Called Dementia, All Problems Become 15

Chapter 6   No Start Button 17

Chapter 7   The Swearing Part Of Your Brain Is The Last To Go 19

Do I Really Need To Know Who The President Is? 20

Chapter 8   How Does A Demented Person Say He's In Pain? 21

Chapter 9   Dementia Language 23

Chapter 10   Strategies 24

How Not To Get Hit When Caring For People Who Have The "Label" Dementia 26

Chapter 11   Love The Caregiver...Especially If It's You! 28

Chapter 12   Dementia And Sex 33

A Final Farewell To My Father 35

Chapter 13   Pastoral Ministry Section* 36

How Not To Get Hit When Ministering To People Who Have The "Label" Dementia 41

Chapter 14   Ladies' Discussion Group 43

Chapter 15   Assessing What Is The First Step? 47

Factors To Check For Prior To Behavior Management 50

Line By Line Suggestions On How To Complete This Form 51

Example Of A Completed Form 55

Behavior Tracking Record 60

Chapter 16   Dementia Language Translator 63

Dementia Self Test* 67

Answer Key 69

Chapter 17   Behavior Management Plans For Care* 71

Index Of Behavior Reasons By Fictitious Person's Name 73

Bibliography: 107

Really Great Books: 109

Free Booklets: 111

Resources For Patients And Families: 113

NO BOOK CAN TAKE THE PLACE OF

AN INDIVIDUALIZED ASSESSMENT

AND RECOMMENDATIONS BY

QUALIFIED HEALTH CARE

PROFESSIONALS.

Since every person with dementia has different symptoms and different impairments, there is no guarantee which approaches will work if any. The purpose of this book is to generate ideas.

GOD Grant Me the

SERENITY

to Accept the Things

I Cannot Change, the

COURAGE

to change the Things I Can, and the

WISDOM

To Know the Difference.

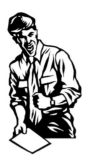

Chapter 1

IN THE BEGINNING

In the beginning my father was able to conceal his confusion from my mother and I by making excuses which at the time seemed reasonable. It wasn't until he told us he was taking pain medication with codeine for his sugar, that we realized he could not remember which pills to take at what time. Then we realized that he was confused. Father had survived lymph cancer and chemotherapy and was considered "in remission." Then we found out he had another type of cancer—colon cancer. We had two days to decide if he would live or die. He had to have a permanent colostomy because the cancer went from a tumor very high in his intestine to a tumor very low, in his rectum. Without the surgery, he would die because he was no longer able to have a bowel movement. So the decision was made. He had to have an permanent ileostomy. We found out much later that he "died" during the surgery. When he died, he was without oxygen long enough to further damage the function of his brain.

Because of the aggressive nature of his cancer, he had to have radiation therapy. As a result of the trauma of his surgery, he became a brittle diabetic for about six months, which for him meant his blood sugar level fluctuated so much we had a great deal of difficulty regulating his insulin. He died and was brought back by paramedics twice because of blood sugar highs and lows. One of the times he died, Mom called the paramedics. I was at work. By the time I got home, there was a message from the nurse on the answering machine. "Debby, you have to come up to the hospital right away, your father needs you." I rushed up to the hospital and Dad said, "Pull the curtain and come here." So I did. He said, "The person in the next bed is crazy." "What?" I responded. He repeated, "The person in the next bed is crazy and I can prove it, look!" He handed me the plastic bag the admissions staff had put his clothing in. On top was the shirt which paramedics had cut into many pieces in order to use the electric heart shock paddles to bring him back to life. He said, "I think he cut up my clothes." I assured him it was the paramedics who cut off his clothes in order to make him better and not to worry, he was safe here. I think this was one of his ways of explaining to me, in the language of dementia, that he no longer understood the world around him.

Dad had to have insulin for the rest of his life. His confusion seemed to worsen noticeably whenever his blood sugar was very high or very low. It was not really his dementia that became worse, but rather, he had become more confused as a result of abnormally high or low blood sugar. When a person is confused due to delirium caused by problems such as low or high blood sugar, dementia behavior management ideas do not work. This is why it is so important to check for medical problems before going to behavior management techniques.

MY BIGGEST LOSS AS A DAUGHTER—

One of the biggest personal losses I experienced from father having dementia was that I could no longer tease him. Because he no longer understood what is normal from what is not normal, teasing him resulted in his acting as though I had hurt his feelings. It was difficult to joke. Dad had always had a wonderful sense of humor and was the world's biggest tease. Up to the day he died, though, if you asked him how he was feeling, he would say, "with my fingers." Unfortunately, confused people can be extremely sensitive to laughter and often interpret teasing as being "laughed at."

THE MOST EMOTIONALLY PAINFUL PART IS <u>WHEN HE KNOWS HE DOESN'T KNOW</u>

The most difficult part of having dementia for father was in the beginning. He knew he was confused. He was so sad. He was constantly trying to figure out what part of his thoughts were correct. It seemed as if he spent the entire day worrying about it and feeling bad. I was almost glad when he became more confused because then he did not realize he was confused! It was less upsetting for him and hence less upsetting for me.

Looking Back...Alzheimer's Took Us by Surprise: (Angela Willis) Looking back on the years I took care of my mother, I realize she hated being dependent. In the beginning of her illness, she knew she was not herself. She recognized her failing memory and inability to think responsibly before anyone in our family was aware of her problem. I believe the physician also initially failed to diagnose her dementia correctly. Diabetes complicated the issue—high and low blood sugars were often given as the reason behind her mood changes, forgetfulness, and inability to sleep at night. Her insulin coverage was adjusted several times, and regular doses were split between the morning and late afternoon. Once the diabetes was stable and her mood swings failed to improve, the physician began to treat her low hemoglobin in the belief that her anemia was causing the behavioral changes. Following blood transfusions and iron therapy, she was still up all night, failed to recognize close friends, and became disoriented in unfamiliar places. She was becoming more restless and also had periods of dizziness where she would fall. (Fortunately, she had no major injuries). Unfortunately, she no longer had the cognition (ability to reason) to identify the cause of her falls, so she could not prevent them. She frequently was found sitting on her buttocks outside the bedroom door or in the middle of the kitchen floor. With the ingenuity to problem solve as only an Alzheimer person can, she'd scoot across the floor on her backside, completely devoid of concern, and with absolutely no clue as to how to get up. After a few such occurrences, I realized she was safer on the floor and decided not to panic about "what it looked like" to my neighbors. She and my youngest son napped together on the living room floor with a pillow, blanket, and the "Days of Our Lives."

She had periods of lucidity, escaping from her imprisoned mind, that were almost frightening to see. She always seemed to know me, but would not remember other family members who were close to her. I remember one time when my older sister came to visit her, she feigned sleep during the entire visit. When the visit was over, she opened one eye and in the voice of a conspirator, she asked, "Is she gone?" I responded, "Yes, but you probably hurt her feelings pretending to sleep." She shook her head and answered, "No, she doesn't really like me."

Another time the parish priest came to visit. The visit was short but congenial. After he left, she asked who he was. She hadn't remembered him; she just knew he was a priest.

Traumatic events were not forgotten and could be easily recalled but were frequently out of context. My niece had a newborn son die and my mother wept passionately for her own infant daughter who died in 1941. For days she spoke about her daughter and the events surrounding her death. She remembered it as if it were yesterday. She became angry at me when I reminded her that it was almost 30 years since my sister had died. Eventually, the memory stopped tormenting her.

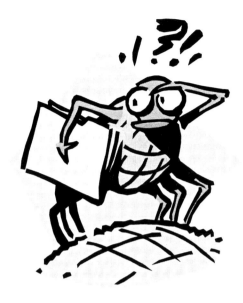

Chapter 2

What Is Dementia?

ALZHEIMER'S DISEASE, ORGANIC BRAIN SYNDROME, DEMENTIA

Alzheimer's disease is a slowly worsening brain disease. It affects more than 4 million Americans (Doka, p. 119). It is marked by changes in behavior and personality and by a decline in thinking abilities. This mental decline is related to a loss of nerve cells and the links between them. Each person is different in the rate at which his or her disease progresses. It advances from mild forgetfulness to severe mental decline. Some warning signs are loss of recent memory, impaired judgment, difficulty doing familiar tasks, problems finding the right words, disorientation to time and place, inability to do simple math, losing things, and personality changes. The person may forget how to do simple things like washing his/her hands, may no longer think clearly or remember words or family members' names (American Alzheimer Assn.). Alzheimer's disease, organic brain syndrome and dementia are terms which are often used interchangeably but I have included the technical definitions for each. I hope these prove helpful to you!

Delirium looks like dementia and the patients may act as though they have Alzheimer's Disease but there are other medical symptoms which, once treated, cause a reverse in the mental status changes. Sudden aggressiveness, also called **acute confusional state** (mental status change) "is a common indicator of acute, treatable illnesses...Delirium is **never a part** of normal aging." (Dept. of Health & Human Services, HCFA; State Operations Manual April 1995, p. 87.)

When mental status change occurs suddenly, often it is delirium but may be diagnosed as dementia because the symptoms are so similar.

"Delirium is often overlooked or unrecognized by many physicians although approximately 50% of patients over the age of 70 on a given medical-surgical unit show some signs of delirium." (Voss-Morice; p. 167.)

Dementia is defined by the 27th Edition Dorland's Medical Dictionary, page 443 as: "A syndrome of progressive decline in multiple areas (domains) of cognitive function eventuallly leading to a significant inability to maintain occupational and social performance."

Delirium is defined by the U. S. Department of Health and Human Services AHCPR publication number 97-0702, page 95 as: "A temporary disordered mental state, characterized by acute and sudden onset of cognitive impairment, disorientation, disturbances in attention, decline in level of consciousness, or perceptual disturbances." **A person can have both dementia and delirium at the same time.**

"Some of the classic signs of delirium may be difficult to recognize and may be mistaken for the natural progression of dementia." (Department of Health and Human Services; State Operations Manual; Provider Certification; Transmittal No. 272; April 1995. p. R-75). When this happens, once the **delirium** is treated (if it can be treated), that person returns to what he or she was like before the problem occurred. If that person were confused before having a urinary tract infection and then suddenly became much more confused (because of the urinary tract infection), the person should return to same level of confusion seen previous to the infection once given antibiotics.

Multi-infarct dementia is defined by the 27th Edition Dorland's Medical Dictionary, page 443 as: "dementia with a stepwise deteriorating course (a series of small strokes) and a "patchy" distribution of neurologic deficits (affecting some functions and not others) caused by cerebrovascular disease."

Organic brain syndrome or organic mental syndrome is defined according to the 27th Edition Dorland's Medical Dictionary, page 1640 as: "DSM III-R includes six specific organic brain syndromes, delirium and dementia; amnestic syndrome or organic hallucinosis; organic delusional syndrome, organic mood syndrome, and organic anxiety syndrome...etc." In other words it is a very generalized word meant to cover many different types of confused behavior, hence not very useful in knowing exactly what type of problem a person may have.

MY FAVORITE DEFINITION OF DEMENTIA: "Dementia is a way of being in the world and separated from one's previous expression of the world."—**Sister Mary Finn, Sacred Heart Major Seminary**

DEMENTIA OF THE ALZHEIMER TYPE Dementia of the Alzheimer type also known as Alzheimer's disease is a progressive neurological and degenerative debilitating brain disorder with major psychosocial and economic repercussions for the victims, their loved ones and society at large (Knopman et al., 2000). This type of dementia afflicts 4 million people. Fewer than 1 victim in 4 receives treatment (Mundt et al., 2000). Alzheimer type dementia occurs slowly and results in memory loss as well as behavior and personality changes. These losses are as a result of the death of brain cells as well as the breakdown of the connections between them. Each victim's course of illness differs as does the rate and symptoms they experience. In normal brain function and aging, brain cells are not lost in great numbers but with Alzheimer type dementia three key processes are disrupted: metabolism, repair, and nerve cell communication. "Two abnormal structures in the brain are the hallmarks of AD: [Alzheimer's Disease] patients live for 8 to 10 years after they are diagnosed, though the disease can last for up to 20 years. AD advances by stages from early mild forgetfulness to a severe loss of mental function. The loss is called dementia." (NIA/NIH, 1999, p.6) Further it is thought that the death of the brain cells may be as a result of amyloid in the brain, formed by the aggregation of fragments which come from a larger protein called APP. If we can understand the way APP functions, we may be able to understand the role of APP in the creation of the amyloid fragments. For example, researchers at the University of California at San Francisco may have found a possible role APP plays in the brain in preventing apoptosis. Apoptosis is a series of cellular events which lead eventually to cell death. This is part of normal functioning, but when this goes wrong it can cause devastating consequences, especially when it occurs in neurons (brain cells) which are irreplaceable. One team of scientists from Harvard Medical School studied two groups of people who died who had been at Massachusetts General Hospital. One group had histories of Alzheimer type dementia and the other group did not. The researchers found that neurites which pass through amyloid deposits in Alzheimer type dementia become twisted and longer than is found in normal brains. The lose their normally straight shape. This lengthening causes delays in the communication between nerve cells. These delays occurring over widespread areas of the brain cause disruption in the cell to cell signaling which is essential for normal cognitive function. (NIA/NIH, 1999)

WHY? In addition, the National Institute of Health scientists are participating in the Brain Molecular Anatomy Project (BMAP) in order to identify and catalog the genes expressed in the nervous system. By making molecular profiles or "fingerprints" of brain cells, scientists will be able to compare gene expression in cells with the clinical state of people and the pathology present in their brain. (NIA/NIH, 1999)

It is estimated that up to 4 million people currently are victims of dementia of the Alzheimer type. Approximately 360,000 new cases will occur each year and this number will increase as the population grows older (Bookmeyer, et al., 1998) "[T]he average lifetime cost per patient is presently $174,000." (Mundt, et al. 2000, p. 163) Most commonly victims of Alzheimer type dementia die of pneumonia. A number of research groups have looked at differences in occurrence in Alzheimer type dementia among racial and ethnic groups. It seems that the risk of getting this type of dementia is higher for African Americans and Hispanic Americans than for Caucasians, although all studies do not agree. The percentage of the non-Caucasian United States population which is over age 65 is estimated to increase from 16 to 34 percent by the year 2050. This fact is important because this disease costs society a lot of money. It is estimated that a victim with Alzheimer type dementia costs between $ 18,408 to $ 36,132 to care for yearly depending on the severity of the impairment. (Leon et al., 1998)

PREVENTION AND TREATMENT

A number of pharmaceutical companies are currently working on 50 to 60 compounds in human trials focusing on treatment for the following three areas:

1) The cognitive decline is currently being treated with a number of drugs which maintain the cholinergic system, such as donepezil which acts to slow down the metabolic breakdown of acetylcholine.

2) Treatment to slow the progress of Alzheimer type dementia, as with anti-inflammatory agents such as prednisone (a steroid) and nonsteroidal anti-inflammatory drugs including ibuprofen, delays its onset or prevents it. Estrogen use has been associated in studies with a decreased risk of Alzheimer type dementia as well as improved cognitive function.

3) Treatments are also being developed for Alzheimer type dementia associated behavior problems. For example, melatonin is a naturally occurring hormone which causes a person to become sleepy; and one study is trying a slow-release melatonin, an immediate-release melatonin, and a placebo to alleviate sleep problems. Non-drug behavior management is also being encouraged. (NIA/NIH, 1999)

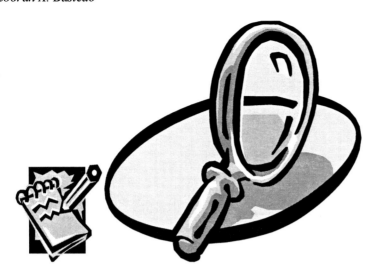

Chapter 3

<u>FACTORS TO RULE OUT PRIOR TO BEING CERTAIN IT IS DEMENTIA</u>
(Sometimes referred to as Mental Status Change.)

The following are common causes for dementia symptoms but may not be dementia. These factors do not include all possible causes.

ISOLATION: Does this person live alone in the country and not go out? Has this person had little people contact, either by choice or by circumstance?

HUSBAND AND WIFE TOGETHER: Each person who has dementia progresses at a different rate and in a different direction. If a husband and wife develop dementia at the same time, it would be unusual. Factors which might cause mental status change for both would need to be evaluated:

- Isolation
- Stressors such as being robbed or conflicts with neighbors
- Contaminated water
- Eating poorly cooked or improperly refrigerated food
- Loss of a loved one (especially husband or wife or child)
- Not eating well
- Not drinking fluids
- Asbestos insulation
- Lead paint
- Slow-leak carbon monoxide
- Communicable disease in the community (Check with local department of public health.)

MEDICAL DISEASE SHOULD <u>ALWAYS</u> BE CHECKED FOR <u>BEFORE</u> A DIAGNOSIS OF ALZHEIMER'S DEMENTIA OR DEMENTIA IS ACCEPTED AS THE PRIMARY CAUSE OF SYMPTOMS. There are many medical reasons why a person can have dementia symptoms even though dementia may not be present.

URINARY TRACT INFECTIONS: One study indicated as much as 83% of the sudden-onset mental status changes seen in the geriatric population are as a result of urinary tract infections. Once an infection is discovered, if the physician treats it and the mental decline reverses, one can conclude the urinary tract infection was the cause. The problem was not primary dementia or Alzheimer's.

RESPIRATORY INFECTIONS - ELEVATED TEMPERATURES, INFECTIONS ANYWHERE IN THE BODY FROM THE TOE TO THE SCALP—ALL CAN CAUSE TEMPORARY MENTAL STATUS CHANGE.

DEHYDRATION: Normal water intake for an adult (with no disease problems which require fluid restriction) is defined as 2500 ml of fluids daily (water or liquids in beverages and water in food). (Dept. of Health & Human Services, HCFA; State Operations Manual April 1995, p. R-55.) However, as we age, our sense of thirst and desire to drink diminishes. Dehydration is a fairly common cause of mental status change, especially in people who live alone. The Federal guidelines which explain to health care inspectors how to interpret the Federal regulations for nursing facilities say our sense of thirst and desire to drink diminishes as we age. Caregivers need to offer water on each contact. I found that when I asked father if he wanted a drink, he would almost always say "no." However, if I put the glass up to his mouth, he would drink. He enjoyed flavored drinks better than water. He liked soda pop best but it would irritate his stomach, so we gave him sugar-free lemonade or sugar-free Kool Aid. According to Quality of Care in Nursing Homes, whenever fluid loss is greater than the amount of fluid taken in then dehydration may occur. According to this book we lose 1500cc as urine and 500-1000 cc through skin and lungs as well as 100cc in feces. (Morris, 332)

MALNUTRITION: According to the Federal guidance to Surveyors of Long Term Care Facilities, p. 107, symptoms of malnutrition include "pale skin, dull eyes, swollen lips, swollen gums, swollen and/or dry tongue with scarlet or magenta hue, poor skin turgor, cachexia, bilateral edema, and muscle wasting." This document considers dementia a risk factor for malnutrition. It further indicates that drug therapy may contribute to nutritional deficiencies including, but not limited to: "cardiac glycosides; diuretics, anti-inflammatory drugs, antacids (if overused), laxatives (if overused), psychotropic drugs (if overused), anticonvulsives, antineoplastic drugs, phenothiazines, oral hypoglycemics as well as poor oral health status or hygiene, poor eyesight, poor motor coordination, or taste alterations (common in dementia), depression or dementia, therapeutic or ground diet, lack of availability of culturally acceptable foods, cancer as well as slow eating." Slow eating or forgetting how to eat is common with dementia.

CONSTIPATION - FECAL IMPACTION: As we age and our body slows, the body's ability to move wastes through the intestinal tract diminishes. It often becomes important for an elderly person to eat a high fiber diet and have a goal of drinking 6 to 10 glasses of water per day.

TUBE FEEDING: On 7-1-95 the Federal government standards for nursing facility practice were amended to include a fluid requirement for all residents, including those on tube feeding which is called enteral (artificial) feeding. Dementia and Alzheimer's persons often become dehydrated because of their failure to drink fluids. Fluids, especially water, have absolutely no appeal for them. Dehydration is one of the major health issues caretakers must deal with. Tube feeding can be through a gastrostomy tube or a nasal tube passed through the nose into the stomach. Tube feeding is often the treatment for dehydration and/or malnutrition which results from the progression of Alzheimer's type dementia.

People on tube feeding need 2500 cc to 3000 cc every 24 hours in order to replace daily what is used daily as well as repair a deficit (Morris, 331) The tube feeding formula will contain 600 to 1000 cc fluid or more, but then additional fluid offered should add up to a minimum of 1500 cc (assuming 1000 cc water in formula). Water must be added before and after each medication. Usually water is also added every 8 hours unless a continuous water added pump is used. The amount needs to be adjusted according to body height as well as number of medications. If the person is receiving a protein supplement to which water is added, this water needs to be counted also. **A registered dietitian should evaluate fluid and formula on the basis of the individual health of the person.**

WARNING: Hospitals usually hydrate patients intravenously (through an IV.) Because of this the 1500 cc instruction for post hospital care is sometimes accidentally left off the transfer information sheet because the water was not needed. The hospital completed fluid requirements with the IV. <u>If your loved one comes home with only</u> tube feeding formula ordered and no IV and no other means of getting water, contact your physician for additional instructions.

PRESSURE ULCERS: True pressure ulcers (also called bedsores) develop from sitting or lying in the same position without changing position. <u>There is a nutritional component to pressure ulcer development.</u> Once pressure ulcers become infected, the infection can cause increased confusion and delirium. Oral antibiotics are an important component of treating an infected pressure ulcer. If not recultured after treatment to determine whether the treatment was effective, the infection can spread through the bloodstream resulting in sepsis which can lead to death. (Dept. of Health & Human Services, HCFA; State Operations Manual, April 1995, p. 88, 157-159.)

Pressure ulcers cannot always be avoided. Alzheimer residents frequently develop anorexia and/or pace excessively, which burns calories faster than they can be replaced. In addition, the need to eat and drink tends to be diminished, which leads to not eating and drinking enough, even without the repetitive behaviors. One continuous 24 hour day of bedrest may result in skin breakdown, depending on the person's health.

SENSORY LOSSES: Sensory impairment (hearing, seeing, taste, touch, smelling) can appear to be dementia because such impairment causes signs of confusion, disorientation, and behavioral changes. Occasionally, this is seen as hallucinations/delusions which are really the person's misinterpretation of noises and images. (Dept. of Health & Human Services, HCFA; State Operations Manual, April 1995, p. 88.) One lady had had her breasts removed prior to admission to a nursing care facility due to cancer of the breast. Unfortunately, she was deaf so she did not understand the explanation the hospital staff gave for surgery. Then when she was transferred to a nursing facility and caregivers approached her she began striking out. How could she know they weren't going to hurt her like she was hurt in the hospital. She was defending herself, not trying to harm anyone.

MEDICATIONS: Medications can cause dementia symptoms to occur. If the change in behavior occurs directly after a change in medication or a new medication, the behavior change could be related to the new medication. Questions one should ask, especially if behavior change is sudden are:

- Is this person on a new medications?
- Could a medication this person has been on have become toxic or have interacted with other drugs?
- Is this person on too many medications?

Drugs which can be a cause of delirium include but are not limited to: antipsychotics; antianxiety/hypnotics, antidepressants; Digoxin/Lanoxin; antiarrhythmics, such as quinidine, Procainamide, Pronestyl, Norpace, calcium channel blockers such as Isoptin (verapamil), Procardia and Cardizem, Inderal and hypertensive medication; gastrointestinal medication such as Tagamet, and Zantac; pain medications -Darvon, morphine, Dilaudid, corticosteroids such as prednisone; anti-inflammatory-Motrin, ibuprofen, cold remedies, sedatives, caffeine, antinausea drugs, alcohol. (Dept. of Health & Human Services, HCFA; State Operations Manual, April 1995, p. 88-89.) Medications can frequently cause an increase in confused behavior. Evaluate and observe behavior as each medication is added. When behavior changes, ask - Is this person on a new medication?

CARDIAC MEDICATIONS: When the physician treats a heart arrhythmia, he may choose to maintain the regular beating of the heart at the cost of mental confusion. One physician explained it to me as a choice—this person could be alive and demented, or dead. I do not think anyone would disagree with this type of logic.

PSYCHOSOCIAL: Recent loss of family or a friend; has the person been robbed, assaulted, or had a serious illness. Restraints, being allowed to remain wet and dirty, being sad or anxious, having a recent change of address (new to current living arrangement = lost) (Dept. of Health & Human Services, HCFA; State Operations Manual, April 1995, p. 89-90).

Recent loss of a loved one or the anniversary date of the death of a loved one may trigger behavioral changes in a person. Grieving is a reaction to the loss. The confused person cannot always pass through the stages of normal grieving because they cannot get beyond the present or the past. The loss stays "trapped" in the person's mind and causes ongoing anxiety. Recognition of this need to grieve can result in providing the help necessary to resolve the unspoken issues.

Fear can trigger changes in behavior which mimic dementia. Has this person experienced a robbery, assault, serious illness, or threat or perceived threat to his or her safety? Fear often appears as paranoia and distrust. Paranoid behavior should be investigated by interviewing family members <u>before</u> a diagnosis of paranoia is given. The fear may be based on facts and exaggerated by circumstances such as living in a new place which appears "strange" due to being unfamiliar.

IS IT DEMENTIA OR IS IT DELIRIUM?

<u>DEMENTIA</u>	<u>DELIRIUM</u>
Slow, progressive brain disorder Occurs over weeks, months, years.	Occurs suddenly, over hours to days.
Gradual change in personality, not always noticed Irreversible.	Usually a sudden change in personality and behavior Usually noticed. Sometimes assumed to be worsening dementia. Potentially reversible.
Involves brain cell death, brain shrinkage.	Usually does not involve brain shrinkage or brain cell death.
Usually does not involve a fever. Cause not always known.	May involve fever, especially low-grade fever. Usually a cause can be identified.
In the beginning, the person knows he is NOT normal and having difficulty.	Usually the person does not realize a problem exists.
Difficulty with simple tasks which he previously could do (can't add, loses things, gets lost)	Reduced clarity of environment (foggy to him).

Delirium can be caused by general medical conditions such as diabetes (high or low blood sugar), urinary tract infections, pneumonia, infections of any kind (skin, toe, decubitus ulcer, upper respiratory infection, etc.), toxic effect of medications, or environmental contamination, or the effect of isolation. ***IT IS POSSIBLE FOR A PERSON TO HAVE DEMENTIA AND DELIRIUM AT THE SAME TIME.*** A person with dementia can have a new problem such as a symptomless urinary tract infection and have delirium symptoms on top of dementia making thinking even less clear and decreasing cognitive and functional abilities.

IS IT DEMENTIA OR IS IT DEPRESSION?

<u>DEMENTIA</u>	<u>DEPRESSION</u>
Sometimes does not sleep long.	Cannot sleep or sleeps too much.
No longer interested in things which he/she used to do a lot.	Loss of interest in things he/she used to do
Anguish because he knows what he knows is not correct (in the beginning of dementia) Things he used to do in 10 minutes now take 2 hours	Sometimes feelings of guilt. Usually loss of energy
Cannot remember recent events Cannot remember things he's always done. Tries to cover up difficulty with memory.	Difficulty concentrating. Memory difficulty. Concerned about difficulty with memory.
Does not remember to eat or eats more often than usual.	Loss of appetite or eats too much.
Slow, progressive brain disorder. Changes in mood noted.	Sometimes slow in beginning. Symptoms may appear suddenly. Mood disorder.
Gradual change in personality not always noticed at first May withdraw & be more quiet.	Tendency to withdraw from people and be more quiet.
Irreversible. Involves brain cell death, brain shrinkage.	Usually potentially reversible. Usually does not involve brain shrinkage.
Neurological symptoms (agnosia - can't remember names, apraxia -can't perform a motor behavior even though muscles capable, aphasia - difficulty with speech) Difficulty with simple tasks which he previously could do.	**NO neurological symptoms.** Reduced clarity of thought.

Depression can be caused by general medical conditions such as diabetes (high or low blood sugar), Parkinson's Disease, Multi-Infarct dementia, death of a significant other, loss of loved ones (often multiple losses), loss of meaningful role in the community, retired no interests, no group of friends, separated from family-too busy, lack of meaningful acitivty, etc.), side effect of medications, chronic pain or the effect of isolation.

OFTEN DEMENTIA AND DEPRESSION OCCUR AT THE SAME TIME. A person with dementia OFTEN has underlying depression which further makes daily life more difficult.

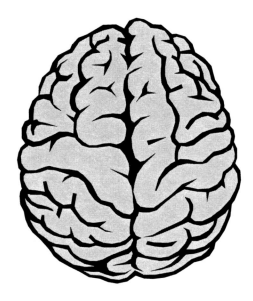

Chapter 4

Why Do They Do the Things They DO?

I'll never forget the time I took my father to the eye doctor and the nurse said about three sentences worth of where to go next. My father looked at me and I said "follow her" in a loud, clear voice to which he replied "okay" and then he did. When using her way of communicating, father couldn't understand what to do. However, when following a simpler dementia way to communicate, he did fine.

IMPAIRED VISION AS AN ACCOMPLICE FOR DEMENTIA The doctor said Dad had a cataract in his left eye. He had the cataract repaired. It wasn't until then that I realized how important eyesight is to a person in understanding his world. At first his vision was a little blurry. After a day or two Dad began looking at everything with great amazement. He would say, "Wow! Look at that sky." Or when we were driving, he would read the signs as we drove. "Wow! 15 feet 6 inches, I never knew the overpass was that high." When I worked with demented people, I noticed that occasionally people who were not able to see very well were referred to a psychiatrist because caregivers would think the confused person's limited vision was evidence of hallucinations. Blurred vision distorts images and may lead to a diagnosis of hallucinations rather than what it is—a distortion or misidentification of shadows as people, or other objects.

One lady told me she thought people were having sex in the hallways at night. Her record indicated she had macular degeneration. When someone has macular degeneration, normal room light makes objects appear to be something they are not. She thought the people walking in the hallway, which were "shadow figures" to her with her diminished vision, were people having sex. The psychiatrist saw her as "delusional" when actually she has impaired vision. After the light bulbs in her room were changed for brighter ones and a night light, her delusions went away. Another lady was given the diagnosis "delusional" because she could not see and her eyes had not been checked. She would "talk to the nurses station," which the psychiatrist thought meant she was "delusional." However, the questions she asked were rational: "Is it time for lunch yet?" "Where am I?" "Why am I here?"

DEAFNESS AS A CO-CONSPIRATOR

One person hit caregivers because she was profoundly deaf but no one had noticed this was the problem. When approached from behind, she would become startled. Her reaction was to hit. Often, in a nursing facility situation, caregivers make it a point to approach profoundly deaf people from the front and touch them gently rather than "grabbing" this person's arm. Grabbing the arm of a deaf person can result in the person swearing and trying to hit the person who grabbed him or her in self defense.

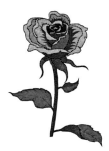

SCRABBLE CONVERSATIONS

My mother-in-law was a very intelligent woman. After she suffered a stroke resulting in a restriction of the blood flow to the brain, talking to her was like playing scrabble. There would be something true about what she was saying but the rest of the words sounded like gibberish. She figured out that when she began speaking in four-word sentences, she could get all four words correct. At first she would say things like, "Go in the kitchen, there's a Domino's pizza there." Then she learned to say, "Check out the fridge." She was trying to communicate that we should help ourselves to something to eat or drink if we wished, but she knew she could not make all the words come out correctly. She knew what she wanted to say. However, it was very frustrating to her when she could not get the words from her brain to her tongue.

When working with people with multi-infarct dementia, I often see such a person swearing or crying or even depressed and refusing to speak. Mom knew what she wanted to say but the words would not come out. Sometimes a person with this type of problem can use a note pad and pen or a picture board or some other method to communicate. When we as caregivers help a person be more independent and feel "normal," more like everyone wants to feel, we have done a lot. Sometimes it is just being patient enough to try to figure out the message.

PLUGGED PLUMBING (Multi Infarct Dementia) COMMUNICATION

Someone with **multi-infarct dementia**, that is someone who has reduced blood flow to the brain, may perceive information in a clogged-sink fashion. The information we try to tell her turns into "confused misinformation," if we use too many words at one time. Just as a clogged sink will have the water spill over the edge if we pour it in too fast, when we try to speak to her with full sentences (normal for everyone else) some of the information "spills over" and she may miss a part of the message.

However, when I:

1. speak clearly and
2. try to keep the message short (4 words are the best)
3. **or** break the message up into parts **and**
4. speak it 4 words at a time and
5. repeat the message several times,

-more of the message gets through more often.

On occasion, my husband and I found we needed to repeat what we were saying over and over. With the first effort, my mother-in-law would get one part of the message; and the next time we said it, she may get the second part. Then during the third or fourth repetition, most of the message would be communicated. Just as with everyone, people with multi-infarct dementia understand better when they are not tired, hungry, or sick.

POWER ISSUES

One of the hardest types of persons to know how to help in a caregiver situation is a person who was accustomed to directing the behavior of other people, especially a man who may have been the president of the company or the immediate supervisor. One woman I met had been a registered nurse and very much resented being "helped." She was notorious for running her wheelchair into people. She voiced frustration over not being able to control her own life. She expressed resentment for "being taking care of." We encouraged her to express her choices and honored them. Rather than just giving her coffee, we would ask her if she wanted coffee. We learned to understand that although she couldn't talk very much, she would rap on her wheelchair tray to indicate she wanted coffee. As long as she felt she had control, she stopped running her wheelchair into people.

One man had run a farm since he was a teenager and had raised two of his wife's brothers, as well as five of his own kids. He also had done volunteer work and was a member of the VFW. Although accustomed to long hours of hard work, at the age of 96 he needed help. Legally blind and hard of hearing he had to depend on others for dressing and bathing; he could not use the bathroom by himself. This man expressed the desire to die. He could give help but did not feel comfortable accepting help.

Another woman, an only child, was accustomed to making choices. She covered up her health problems and went into an apartment living situation which included a nursing facility as part of the complex. Prior to that she could not see very well and had to give up driving. She had severe osteoporosis and had had her right hip pinned. Her legs would collapse and she would fall but she did not tell anyone. One day during a fire drill, she fell and broke her hip. It turned out her hip bone had collapsed due to its weakened bone structure.

"NO" IS A POWERFUL WORD

Men who have dementia like to say "NO" when caregivers ask them to do something or cooperate with care. Father would look at us and say, "I said NO" as loud as he could. One nurse said she thought her father tried to ask questions to which caregivers would say NO because he liked the feeling of power he had when he yelled at them. When she did say NO, he would become angry and start swearing. By becoming angry, he felt he was making choices, having some control over a world which he no longer understood. One idea is to try to answer him in a way which would not include NO, so that he would not need to blow up and become angry. For example, if he says he wants to go to town, the caregiver can reply, "Yes, I know you want to go to town, but now is not a good time." Another time when "no" is used as a power word is when bathing is involved. One way I found of avoiding this confrontation was to avoid discussing bathing and simply put Dad in the tub. Usually he would be halfway done before he realized what was happening. Another method was to ask him if he wanted his bath now or in 15 minutes. That way, he got a chance to choose.

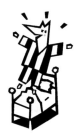

Chapter 5

ONCE CALLED DEMENTIA, ALL PROBLEMS BECOME...

Many times, I note psychological consultations being ordered before reviewing symptoms in order to see if other problems could be causing the symptoms or making the person's confusion worse. Caregivers need to make sure the physician is made aware of the current problems and identified changes. This is especially important when a sudden change in behavior is noted. When treating demented residents, this type of information becomes increasingly important. I have seen patients who were classified as having Alzheimer-type dementia miraculously lose their dementia once a urinary tract infection or imbalance in their blood was treated. I developed forms (they can be found in this book.) for use in screening out other potential reasons for confused behavior. In addition, the following information is from the requirements of the Federal Conditions for Participation for nursing homes:

The Federal regulation for this is on page 127 of the HCFA Guidelines for participation in Medicaid for nursing homes, which states, in part: "The resident's physician provides a justification **why** the **continued use** of the drug **and the dose** of the drug **is clinically appropriate.** This justification should include:

(a) a diagnosis, but not simply a diagnostic label or code, but the description of symptoms,
(b) a discussion of the differential psychiatric and medical diagnosis (e.g., why the resident's behavioral symptom is thought to be a result of a dementia with associated psychosis and/or agitated behaviors, and **not** the result of <u>an unrecognized painful medical condition</u> or a psychosocial or environmental stressor),
(c) a description of the <u>justification for the choice</u> of a particular treatment, or treatments, and
(d) a discussion of <u>why the present dose is necessary</u> to manage the symptoms of the resident. This information need not necessarily be in the physician's progress notes, but must be a part of the resident's clinical record."

FURTHER, when the Federal government developed the instruction manual for the minimum assessment data required for each nursing facility resident, the Resident Assessment Instrument (Minimum Data Set or MDS), the Health Care Financing Administration adopted the following identification criteria which I have paraphrased for your benefit:

Factors to consider for MOOD changes which are not necessarily related to dementia:

<u>Depression symptoms</u> -> Some symptoms are *weight loss, weight gain, crying, tearfulness, agitation, aches and pains, withdrawal from normal activity pattern, decline in ability to do or assist with activities of daily living.* Depression can cause such decline. Such decline can also cause depression.

<u>Recent Life Changes</u> -> Such as the *death of loved one,* roommate, friend, caregiver, new admission to nursing facility or assisted or supervised apartment. Has there been *a separation from loved ones,*

functional loss of ability, change in body image (such as new colostomy), loss of independence? How long ago did this occur? Is the mood change normal as a result of a recent loss or a problem as a result of this person being unable to adjust to a loss from 10 years ago? *Is the behavior change part of a pattern or cycle which may relate to existing disease.* Is there ***a new problem*** which may be the cause?

Is there a <u>communication decline</u>? Is this person <u>hard of hearing</u>? Does this person misunderstand his or her environment because of severe **visual difficulty**, such as the person who told me her caregivers were having sex in the hallway. The shadows she saw looked like people having sex to her.

According to the Federal guidelines, rather than assess this person for psychiatric drugs, one would want to <u>try increasing the number of watts of lighting and maybe providing better glasses if possible</u>. The guidelines further suggest useful strategies of modifying the environment, **separating activities of daily living into smaller tasks** and <u>using verbal reminders</u> or cues as to the next step. Further information from the Federal Guidelines for nursing facility care indicate we should <u>evaluate metabolic causes</u> for mood changes such as *electrolyte imbalance, dehydration, respiratory causes, high or low blood sugar, urinary tract infection, constipation, infection anywhere in body, reduced blood flow to the brain*, etc.

Take **extra care to identify people who are passive and quiet** who might otherwise be overlooked. *Conditions listed which can affect mood: Alzheimer's disease, cancer, stroke or other neurological problems, cardiac, metabolic (Addison's disease, low blood sugar, high blood sugar), endocrine (hypercalcemia, hyperthyroidism, Cushing's disease).* "Further, using **some medications can cause decline in mood** such as

> clonidine (Catapres)
> guanethidine (Ismelin)
> methlydopa (Aldomet)
> propranolol (Inderal)
> Reserpine
> cimetidine (Tagamet)   cytoxic agents
> Digitalis   immunosuppressives
> sedatives   steroids
> and stimulants.

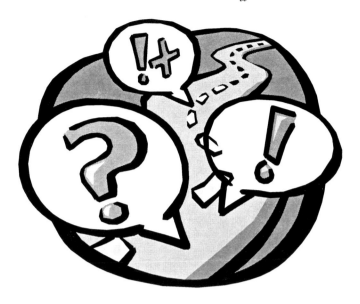

Chapter 6

NO START BUTTON

Beth Spencer, MSW, one of the co-authors of Understanding Difficult Behavior, once explained to me that having Alzheimer-type dementia is like losing your start button. That is, you lose your ability to remember how to begin activities. I think this may be one reason why simple day-to-day tasks which take a non-dementia person 15 minutes may take Alzheimer-type dementia people two hours or even an entire day. Once I came upon a man with Alzheimer's who had tipped over a small table. He bent over to pick it up but could not remember the next step was to grab the table, then pick it up. Instead of picking up the table for him, I put my arms around him, then gently lowered his hands and we grasped the table together and lifted it upright. He gave me a very heartfelt, "THANK YOU!" I felt as though I had helped someone scratch an itch under a cast because there was such a tremendous sense of relief to his thank you.

One person with Alzheimer-type dementia had taken off his shirt. He just stood there holding his shirt. I helped him place his arms in the shirt and buttoned the first button. He could not button the first button but once I did, he could button the rest. It was like he did not have a second-step or what to do next button but once a task was started, he could keep going and maybe even finish it.

Some people with this type dementia can do tasks if we give them step-by-step directions. Some people cannot. Just as each person has a unique set of genes and chromosomes and culture and family history, each person does dementia his or her own way.

I notice that when in a strange place or noisy place, or if furniture is moved around, or if there are a lot of boxes or the normal environment is not like it usually is, people with dementia become more mentally impaired. They strike out or become verbally abusive.

One of the easiest problems to miss relating to this confusion is when a person cannot remember all the steps when eating. One day he can feed himself; the next day he sits there and appears to be eating but none of the food is actually being swallowed. I have seen people stir their food and pick up a spoonful, put it back down and stir their food and pick it up. They may place a spoonful of food in their mouth and store it in their cheeks without actually swallowing anything. One person in particular with Alzheimer-type dementia would pick up food from his tray but never actually put it into his mouth. He would move his napkin and straighten his tray but never actually eat anything. Occasionally this change in status is identified only when a dramatic weight loss has occurred. One solution is to stand next to the person to remind him step by step how to eat.

Some demented people cannot eat in a dining room with other people or cannot eat if company comes over. Dad went through periods when he could not eat unless he was sitting at the table with no distractions. If anybody spoke to him, he lost track of what he was doing and would stop eating. If the television or a radio were playing, he could not remember what to do. When he first came home from the hospital after his colostomy, I would offer him a snack before bedtime. He would always say, "No." Then he would sit at the dining room table and put his napkin to his chin. I learned to understand this daily "No" as a "Yes" in the language of dementia.

We need to make sure to watch a confused person to make certain he or she is eating. If not eating, then try to empower that person by beginning his feeding, then letting him/her take over. Place the spoon in his hands. See if he can complete the activity. If you eat with him sometimes he can mimic what you do, even though on his own he does not remember what to do next. Caregivers need to encourage the person to drink each time they encounter him in order to encourage hydration. I found that I was more successful getting my father to drink if I talked about something else and just placed the cup to his lips. One of the things I learned about getting him to do things was to offer alternatives which both meant the same thing. His "NO" always worked better and faster than his ability to understand what I was really saying. I'll never forget when he came home from the hospital after just having had his colostomy (1989.) He never did like bathing in winter because when he was a kid his family thought people got pneumonia from taking baths in the winter. If you asked his permission first, he would never have had another bath, or shower. Just like my kids when they were two years old, "NO" was his favorite word. His caregiver would talk about something else or say, "What is your favorite, tub bath or shower?" He got so he would begin conversations with "I'm not taking a shower today, I've already had one." At this point the caregiver would talk about world news or a relative he remembered, take his hand and talk and walk to the bathroom. If the conversation was interesting enough, he would be halfway done before he realized what we were doing.

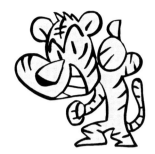

Chapter 7

THE SWEARING PART OF YOUR BRAIN IS THE LAST TO GO

Before becoming confused, father did not swear very often. After he became confused, however, and the more confused he became, the better he got at swearing. I read an article one time which said that dendrites (brain cell nerve fibers) continue to grow as we age. The article continued to say these cells reconnect to older cells just as the more recent memory cells become disconnected. That is why people remember things in the past better than recent events. It is also why people with dementia forget words they've remembered for years. Swearing becomes a way of expressing frustration over knowing what you want to say but not being able to remember the words.

The most frequent reason I see confused people swear is because they cannot think of the words they are trying to say. The swearing actually represents frustration more than the meaning of the actual word. When father would begin swearing, I would try to get him to talk about something else, something he could remember and distract him in that way. Another reason I saw him swear was if he thought something was going to hurt such as a bed bath. Toward the end of his life, he had lost so much weight that just touching him would hurt. The day before he died I touched his shoulder to kiss him as I was going to work and his shoulder went "crack." I cannot help but believe it hurt. We could not keep from touching him, but smiling, making eye contact, and talking to him in a gentle, happy voice helped him not be afraid. It was hard when we were in public such as going to the doctor's office. I finally developed the technique of looking at people who were sworn at and, using my happiest voice, I would say, "The swearing part of your brain is the last to go." Then I would talk about something else (distracting and changing the subject sometimes works for people who are not confused, too). Sympathizing with the person who is swearing, especially if you know why he or she is swearing can be very comforting to them.

Caregivers need to be aware of changes in the Alzheimer dementia person's response to everyday situations. Every episode of "acting out" may not be an expression of dementia but may relate to a new problem. For example, a failure to eat breakfast may not be stubbornness, but a sore throat. *A person with dementia cannot usually put a name on his discomfort, but acts it out instead.* Be aware of **facial expressions** as well as changes in energy level. If you have a headache from being up all night with mom or dad, maybe he or she does too. If the chili at supper upset your stomach, maybe it upset mom's or dad's stomach also. Look for non-verbal clues to problems. Every behavior change is not "just Alzheimer's."

DO I REALLY NEED TO KNOW WHO THE PRESIDENT IS?

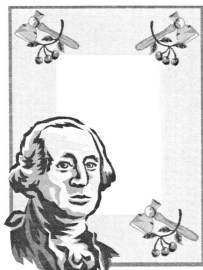

One of the things I notice when working with confused people is that looking them in the eye and talking to them like they are normal <u>makes them more normal</u>. The person often acts as though it is such a relief to be viewed as a normal person. One sad and tearful gentleman came up to me and said, "My wife is dead and I don't know what to do." I looked him in the eye and said, "Your wife is fine, she came to visit you yesterday." He replied, "Is my daughter okay, too?" I said, "Yes, she came to visit you yesterday, too." He said, "Oh, I'm so glad, I thought she was dead. Did I tell you I was in the war." His mood changed to a happy one and we could then discuss other things. We decided to keep a notebook in his room where his wife and daughter would sign in when they came to visit to let him know that they are still alive.

Whenever doctors or nurses would evaluate Dad's confusion, they would ask him the name of the President. He would wrinkle his brow and do his best to think of a President's name. One day it would be President Truman, the next it would be President Carter. Daddy almost never got this one right, and it always bothered him. He might name about six of them and watch the person's face to see if any answer was correct. Then he would knit his brow and get that look people get when they have more bills than paychecks. One of the questions I asked myself when taking care of my father was, "Does he really need to know who the President is?" My answer was "no." The value of a person is much more than what that person can memorize. I treated dad with love and continued to value that part of my father which I could still recognize as I saw his confusion become worse. Because it bothered him when people asked him that question and he would get it wrong, I would say, "It's okay Daddy, he just raised our taxes, it's better not to know."

"It's okay" became one of my favorite phrases to use. I could always tell when he was worried because he would knit his brow. We wouldn't even be talking and he would sit there with a worried expression on his face. So I would say, "What are you worried about?" He would say, "I don't know how I'm going to pay my bills." I would say, "Don't worry, we paid ahead" or "It's my turn to worry, you already had your turn." "It's okay." Then I would change the subject and try to get him to "un-worry." I could tell if he was worrying by whether he had furrows on his forehead. I see this in other confused people too. Telling him or her "it's okay" or "don't worry" seems to make him or her feel a little better.

When near the confused person, the caregiver should be noticing how this person looks and acts. Caregivers need to be like Sherlock Holmes and watch for changes in behavior or "acting out" which will help identify additional problems or needs. Because people with dementia are confused to some degree, new symptoms are often seen as "just Alzheimer's" rather than looking for the reason the person is acting this way.

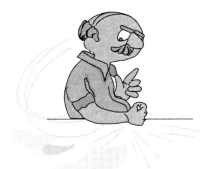

Chapter 8

HOW DOES A DEMENTED PERSON SAY HE'S IN PAIN?

A demented person, when approached for a bath or for clothing changes, may start yelling and try to hit the caregiver. I see this as evidence of existing or "anticipated" pain. We had a home health Certified Nursing Assistant (CENA) who would come to give father a bath. She reached for his arm. Before she touched it, he would start hollering, "It hurts, it hurts." She said, "But David, I did not touch you yet." In the language of dementia, he was telling us that moving him hurt because his bones were brittle and he had arthritis. He was expecting pain. Probably he already was in some pain but could not tell us.

DEMENTED WAYS TO SAY "I'M IN PAIN!"

1. Crying or tearfulness (When asked will say, "No, I'm not in pain")
2. Restless - unable to hold still
3. Hitting caregivers (or trying to hit them)
4. Swearing, especially if very loud
5. **Resisting, refusing to allow caregivers help change his clothes, bathe, or help the person move from one place to another
6. Saying over and over things which sound like pain- "I hurt, I hurt"
7. "Throwing" himself because having been in the same position for so long, he cannot say he hurts and needs to escape the pain. Sometimes the x-ray will show compressed vertebrac.
8. Unable to find a comfortable position in bed; the person does not sleep but instead paces and repeatedly gets out of bed.
9. Quadriplegics who "throw" themselves across the room because they are in the same position in their chair for too long and cannot tell you they hurt; often there will be an x-ray indicating vertebral disc compressions or severe bone degeneration— osteoarthritis
10. Pained facial expressions.
11. Taking clothing off - especially if the person takes all clothing off. (can be constipation, hemorrhoids, abdominal pain, rectal itching, etc.)
12. Pained facial expression, esp. grimacing, or knitting eyebrows.
13. Drawing up knees to chest (fetal position).
14. Writhing in the bed.
15. Trying to escape the building in order to escape the pain.
16. Urinating in his/her pants in wheelchair next to toilet (transferring from the wheelchair onto the toilet seat hurts).
17. Refusing therapy - physical therapy, occupational therapy, or other care, etc.

18. Self consoling behavior such as rocking back and forth.
19. Threatens other people, very angry.
20. Throwing objects.
21. Refuses to eat because of tooth ache but he cannot tell you it hurts.
22. Grabbing the caregivers arm very hard and refusing to let go.
23. Expressing the desire to die, "I can't take this anymore!"

SOLUTIONS:

If you give a demented person a pain medication and the behavior stops then you know for sure it was pain.

The best solution is to change the environment, in bed and in wheelchair get positioning pillows.

Preventive pain Medication BEFORE therapy, especially physical therapy - it almost always hurts.

One lady in a wheelchair would wheel up to the toilet and even though she could transfer to the toilet, she would urinate in the wheelchair. We solved this problem by getting her a raised toilet seat so she didn't have to bend down so far to sit on the toilet.

Try to avoid assisting with transfer using armpits or shoulders, often shoulders have arthritis or injury making this a painful area for this person.

Allow him or her to take your hand.

Allow him to help. Sometimes if you let him hold an empty razor, he will sit patiently and allow the caregiver to shave him.

Don't grab the person, unless it is an emergency situation, let him or her take your hand.

In late stage dementia primitive reflexes return, esp. **"Paratonia"** which is the involuntary resistance in a leg or arm to a sudden passive movement. (Kovach, 8) With this type of reflex the person is not even trying to hit someone, it is a reflex. This means that if you grab a demented person, they will hit you if they have reached this stage in the disease.

ENVIRONMENTAL MODIFICATION: People who have dementia need an around-the-clock activities area where they have objects to manipulate and things to occupy their attention. They need distraction but not necessarily noise as many cannot tolerate confusion and noise. A regular schedule with events following the same order every day. This lessens fear and makes the environment more comfortable. They need to have the environment modified for them. That is, if their vision is poor, they may need to have higher watt light bulbs and/or a brightly colored or glow-in-the-dark toilet seat so they can find the toilet. Beth Spencer told me she had one man who would urinate everywhere except the toilet until she wrote "TOILET" in big two-inch letters and placed it above the toilet.

Some people need their picture or their name on their bedroom door because they cannot remember which room is theirs. They may go into the wrong room and go to bed. They even will crawl in bed with someone else. I have seen caregivers place a drawing of a toilet on the bathroom door to help a demented person find the bathroom. This may help prevent the person from urinating in the wastebasket in other rooms.

A raised toilet seat may help others to use the toilet. The chief benefit of a raised toilet seat is that if you have arthritis, you do not have to sit so far down and it does not hurt as much to use it. A demented person may not be able to tell you it hurts when he or she uses the toilet. Instead, being wet or not "making it" to the toilet may be a demented way to say, "Using the toilet hurts!"

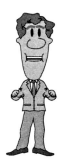

Chapter 9

DEMENTIA LANGUAGE

"I WANT TO MAKE CHOICES"

To me, dementia is like not having a "frame" around one's world. Dad could not remember who the President was, what day it was, or other basic information which gives each of us a feeling of control over our lives. Each of us takes for granted the fact that we "know" what day it is, what time it is, what to do next, how to get dressed, how to add numbers. When Dad was in the early stages of dementia, he would try to "empower himself" by taking some control over life. He would become demanding over what he seemed to feel were the choices he <u>could</u> make. For example, he always liked to go somewhere in the car. We would take him to the gas station when we filled up the gas tank. He liked one specific gas pump. If we went to any other station or any other pump at the station he liked, he would swear and carry on like crazy. At first it was irritating to have to wait in line for our turn at the "correct" pump when there were other pumps not in use. But after a while, I thought it was cute. I found that if I allowed him to have control over things that did not matter (like which gas pump to use), he would cooperate better with me when I wanted him to do something.

I NEED A FRAME AROUND MY WORLD

When a confused person insists on caregivers acknowledging his or her interpretation of the world, he is really saying there is no frame around his world. No matter how silly I think what he is saying "sounds like," it is his way of putting a frame around his world. He was trying to fill in the blanks in a world where he did not know what day it was. He did not know what time it was. He did not know the President's name. To me it was like he needed to be correct about **one** thing he believed whether it was correct or not. It was almost as if agreeing with **one thing** made everything else which seemed too confusing to him somehow make sense.

IF YOU CAN'T WIN THE BATTLE -CHANGE THE WAR

It did not take long for me to learn that the best way to avoid getting hit, bitten, or threatened and to avoid swear words was to change the war. I learned to redirect father's behavior by changing the subject. I knew he would not give up about whatever his mind was focused on, but I could ask him something else or change the subject. He would tend to come back to the thought his mind was focused on but I might get 15 minutes of peace by changing the subject. I might ask him what he thought about it and then let him talk. What he said may not make sense to me, but even demented people need to talk. It is part of being human. It seemed to make him feel better, just as it makes me feel better to talk about my problems with my friends.

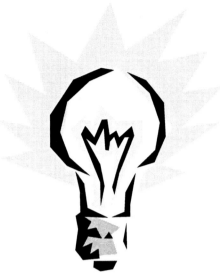

Chapter 10   STRATEGIES

DON'T ARGUE

Arguing with ANY confused person is more apt to get you hit, bit, kicked or hurt. Father knew his world but he no longer understood the world of regular "undemented" people. His world (dementia interpreted) was just as real to him as our world is to us. Once he insisted there were spacemen in orange suits in an apple tree outside the window of his hospital room. Whenever I tried to tell him he was on the fifth floor of the hospital, he would insist there were spacemen. He would say, "Can't you see the spacemen in the orange suits?" When I honestly replied, "No," he became very angry and started swearing. Since I did not want to cause more trouble, I agreed there were orange spacemen. He calmed down. During this period of his confusion, he would sit in the hospital room and "watch the wall move." He had just had major surgery and his blood sugar was not in balance. I am sure he was delirious, but he still needed to have validation for his viewpoint of the world. Naomi Feil is a certified activity director who wrote a book entitled The Validation Breakthrough. I understand her approach is to repeat what the confused person is saying so that person can let it go. My mother refused to agree with anything dad said if it was incorrect which did not help and made him angrier. She argued with Dad about everything. He responded by hitting at her, screaming and/or swearing loudly. He would become so upset that I worried he would burst a blood vessel in his head! My approach was to allow Dad to have his world. I did not argue with him but rather tried to nudge him in the right direction. He never once hit me. It is your decision as a caregiver as to the approach you use. To me Dad was more important than the name of the President. If it made him happy to see orange spacemen, then orange spacemen were okay with me, too.

GIVE HIM SOMETHING TO HAVE AND TO HOLD

When we left the house, Father became more confused. I believe it related to home feeling "familiar" and having a sense of knowing what to expect. When Father had a urinary tract infection, he had to be admitted to the hospital for treatment. After a few days, it was time to take him home. First, he had to change out of his hospital gown and into street clothes. This may not sound too challenging but he had a colostomy (an opening in the abdominal wall, to which a bag is attached, to handle solid body waste when the rectum is surgically removed) and a bladder catheter. In addition, since he wasn't at home, everything was more confusing to him and he was less able to help. When he could not understand his environment, he changed his focus to the catheter and the colostomy and would begin to fuss or tug on them. Sometimes he would cause them to leak or come off, which would soil him and his clothing and greatly increase the amount of time needed to get him ready. I felt I could either spend two hours getting him dressed OR I could give him something to hold. I knew that he would not be able to both tug at his colostomy or catheter and hold his hat. I gave him his hat and said, "Dad, you better hang onto this hat so we don't forget it." He dutifully held it for about five minutes, after which he put it on his head and began reaching for his "tubes." I knew from past experience that if I did not do something, he would either pull out his catheter or rip off his colostomy bag. Searching for something else I could give him to hold, I noticed he had not eaten his apple at lunch. I gave him the apple to hold, which he did hold with both hands. When he would start to set it down, I would remind him Mom would be angry if he wasted good food and that he should hang onto it. He did. I had him dressed in 10 or 15 minutes and we were on our way. If I had had to wrestle with him over his tubes it would have probably taken more than an hour.

DO MAKE EYE CONTACT - TREAT HER WITH RESPECT

All people want to be treated with respect. One of the most important ways to reach a demented person is to "look her in the eye." Although a confused person may appear to be speaking "gibberish," one does not know if this is because of confusion, being hard of hearing, or a malfunction of the brain in communicating. I DO know that I always look the person in the eye. This accomplishes two important objectives. One, it makes that person "feel" more "normal." Two, it communicates respect and makes contact with her. One of the most interesting things which tends to happen when making eye contact is that the person will make more sense. I have literally had demented people go from "gibberish" to real words, just by making eye contact with them and being patient and waiting for them to finish.

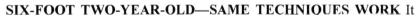

SIX-FOOT TWO-YEAR-OLD—SAME TECHNIQUES WORK It may sound disrespectful for an adult child to see his or her demented parent as a six-foot 2-year-old; however, I found the same behavior management techniques work for the very young and the very old. For example, if we went out, I took an adult version of a diaper bag with tape and bandages and colostomy supplies. If father got upset over being in a strange place, and ripped off his colostomy bag, we would have a way to replace it. Mom or I would carry his medications as well as hard candy just in case he got faint or pale or more confused, indicating low blood sugar. We also carried a change of clothes because he could accidentally get himself all wet trying to use the toilet (just like a 2-year-old).

When we had to wait in the doctor's office or elsewhere, I would try to have a couple of magazines or something I could hand him to look at so he would not get in trouble. He found it difficult to sit and wait. He didn't watch television because he was unable to follow the plot, although he did like to look at the picture occasionally. Instead of spending the entire 30-minute to 60-minute wait walking him back from the door, I diverted his attention by giving him something else to think about and handing him magazine after magazine. I could hand him the same magazine more than once, he didn't remember he had seen it.

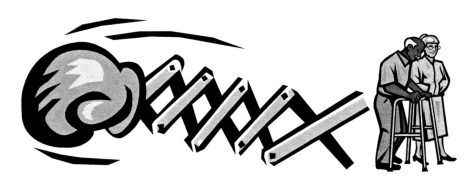

HOW NOT TO GET HIT WHEN CARING FOR PEOPLE WHO HAVE THE "LABEL" DEMENTIA

1. Make **eye contact**, <u>wear a pleasant expression</u> on your face. A simple **"hello"** spoken with affection can mean more than volumes of conversation.
2. **Keep the conversation simple**, use simple words, see how the person reacts, then try to speak to her at her level of understanding.

DO NOT "TALK ***DOWN***" TO THE PERSON. She STILL has feelings which can be hurt. If the person does not appear to be understanding your words, then 2 possible causes can be:

    a. **Hard of hearing**? Try using words on paper - or pointing - touch her gently to provide reassurance or gesture.
    b. Dementia may be related to clogged arteries in the brain (multi-infarct dementia is one label). <u>Only part of what you are saying may be heard:</u>
        i) **speak louder and clearer**
        ii) **use simple words**
        iii) **use 4 word sentences** such as "follow me, this way" rather than "if you will follow me, we will go to the main dining room." (too many words to understand)

    c. **Repeat your 4 word sentence several times** as each time that person may get a little more of the message. It is like plugged plumbing. If you try to pour a bucket of water down a stopped sink fast, you will end up spilling water over the edge of the sink. But if you pour water a little at a time, eventually it will all go down the drain.

3. **Try not to startle the person**, or grab her. Try not to put the person in a situation with too much noise or where there is too much background activity or noise. <u>The more noise and activity there is, the more the demented person's ability to understand will diminish.</u>
4. **Change the subject.** If this person continues to "focus" her thoughts on one concept (such as "My mother needs me home to do the dishes."), ask about her mother **or try to repeat what she is saying;** then change the subject. "Oh, your mother needs you home to do the dishes. You must be a good daughter; what is your mother like?"
5. <u>DO NOT ARGUE WITH THIS PERSON.</u> There is no better way to get hit than to argue. She needs to know you accept her as she is.
6. **Do not try to "force" the person to do something. Instead suggest 1 or 2 alternatives** and ask which she would like. (*DO NOT OFFER AN ALTERNATIVE WHICH WOULD ENCOURAGE HER TO DO WHAT SHE IS ATTEMPTING TO DO WHICH IS NOT OKAY.*) For example, "I want to go home, right now." Say, "Oh you want to go home right now, but I came to visit you. Should we go to the dining room or the day room?" Or ask her to tell you about "home" AND why she wants to go there.

7. **When a person has dementia, being treated with respect and dignity becomes increasingly important.** Respect can allow someone with Alzheimer's dementia to do more than she reasonably should be able to do, because it is expected of her. People tend to rise to the level of our expectations. If we expect nothing, that is what this person will accomplish. Sometimes the frustration of this can lead to combative behavior.

WHAT IF THE PERSON DOES BECOME COMBATIVE?

<u>Try not to put yourself in a situation where you are 'cornered.'</u> I had a 6-foot 5-inch very strong demented person corner me in a room. He then began to come after my throat with his hands. There was no door or window except behind him. One of the things a person loses when they get dementia is his or her inhibitions relating to inappropriate behavior. This person is not necessarily mentally ill. I just think of it as though his brain were a switchboard with some of the wires connected wrong.

Look to see what he or she was doing directly before becoming difficult and try to avoid that happening again.

For example, once when Mom and I took Dad out to eat at a restaurant, he looked at the menu and started swearing and took a swing at my Mom. What was the trigger for the behavior? The menu—too many hard choices, too complicated. **His anger was a reaction to the frustration of not being able to figure out what to do.**

After that, we learned to:

1) Do not give him a menu.
2) Do not argue with him.
3) Offer him two choices.

He would say, "What do I want to eat?" To which we would reply, "Today you're in the mood for meatloaf and coffee." He would then say, "That sounds good."

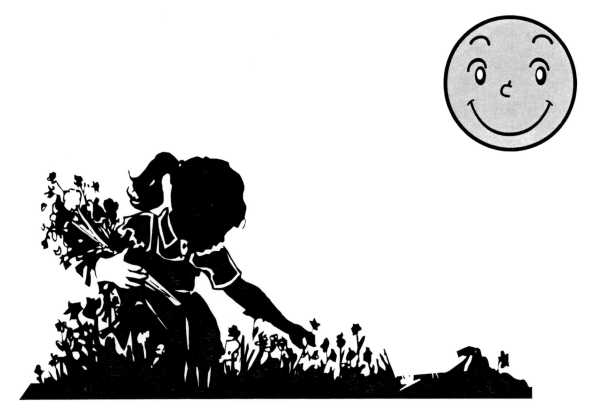

Chapter 11

LOVE THE CAREGIVER...ESPECIALLY IF IT'S YOU!

There is no harder role than the role of the caregiver. Everyone's attention is focused on the demented person. The caregiver is overlooked. Try to do something special for you. Get help. Take time to go to a movie or read by having someone watch him or her for you. No one should make themselves a martyr constantly caring for a demented person. The most tragic thing I have ever seen is a son who died of a heart attack taking care of his mom who did not recognize him. She then went on to live in a nursing facility where she does well; however, she is still waiting for her son's visit. If he had taken her to the nursing facility when the burden became too great, or if he had gotten help such as respite caregivers, he might still be alive to visit his mother and enjoy his time with her. No mother wants to be a burden to her child.

FIND THE MAGIC IN EACH DAY

Even though it is very hard to deal with the constant needs of a demented person, I found I did better if I tried to find "some magic" in each day. The magic may be watching the birds or smelling the flowers, or in enjoying something "cute" Father had done. I know it is hard to see some of the things a demented person does as cute; however, I thought of Dad affectionately as a six-foot 2-year-old and tried to enjoy him from that perspective. After becoming demented he could not get his hair combed in a way it would look good. He went around with a cow lick group of hairs sticking straight up like Dennis the Menace. I found it difficult not to think of him as cute with this haircut.

DON'T BLAME THE NURSING FACILITY

We must remember that in a nursing facility caregivers are assigned to several people -not just one. While we may see only what Father cannot do, we often miss the fact that such caregivers have kept Dad alive. Many bad things have not happened due to staff watching over him. I know some of the newspapers love to bash nursing facilities, especially when there are no new scandals. Many of the most loving, caring people I have ever met work at nursing facilities. In order to work at a nursing facility, you have to be willing to accept abusive language and be ready to duck, literally. You have to submit to multiple highly critical surveys from both the state and Federal regulatory agencies. Nursing facilities are the black sheep of the health care industry. Everyone likes to complain and criticize but so few people are willing to volunteer to help. Research indicates 95% of all abuse occurs <u>at home</u>, not in nursing facilities (Comer p. 703.) If you do not like the nursing facility where your loved one stays, go in, volunteer and make it a better place to live. There are so many people who live there that do not have family or do not have visitors. Make somebody's day! Go and visit a nursing facility resident! It won't hurt. You may even feel better.

CAREGIVER ANGER AND FRUSTRATION

It is okay to be angry. It is okay to <u>want</u> to hit him or her. It is NOT okay to <u>actually</u> hit him or her.

Someone who cares for a demented person has <u>every right to become angry</u>. It is a very frustrating situation to be in. We need to stop short of harm. I "lost it" and yelled at father on more than one occasion; but I really tried not to because it wasn't his problem but my frustration. Anger breeds anger. People with dementia are more easily "pushed" into anger. I found it far easier to work with Dad if I did not argue. One of my friends who cared for her Alzheimer mom was in tears. When I asked her what was wrong, she said, "I yelled at her. She did not understand and I yelled at her!" No one can change the past but each of us can try other ways in the future. The great thing about having a poor memory is that that person will not remember you yelled. Please know that if you didn't lose it once in a while, you wouldn't be human. Each day is an opportunity to do better than the day before—start over, manage the behavior; then you won't have to feel guilty.

DO YOUR BEST—IT'S OKAY

I think of the time I spent with father, and I know I did some things wrong. The fact that we are each human results in each of us making mistakes. I tried to use the Cub Scout motto, "Do your best!" I know I did the best I could under very difficult conditions. And you should know the same about you.

SOMETIMES DENIAL IS OKAY

Mother denied Father had Alzheimer's from the day the doctor told us and she still denies it today. I think it is easier for her to cope this way. There is nothing wrong with that. She said, "He just does these things to give me a hard time and make life more difficult." Surprisingly, the fact that she expected him to do for himself seemed to keep him independent longer. <u>The fact that she repeated what she expected him to do over and over helped direct him</u>. They would fight and scream at each other. To a certain extent this actually provided an emotional vent for them both. I finally convinced Mom to stop arguing, because Dad would get so mad he would hit her. She had many bruises as a result.

PLAN REST TIME FOR YOURSELF—LOCK THE BATHROOM DOOR

We have a whirlpool tub and since I have severe degenerative arthritis, I like to sit in it when I am really sore. One problem, however, was that if I did not remember to lock the door, Dad would come in to be with me. The bathroom was his favorite place anyway. Having someone to talk to was wonderful for him. Eventually, I learned to lock the bathroom door so I had at least one hour of peace. Dad was fine. I felt better.

IT IS OKAY TO LET GO AND GET HELP

Each of us has a number of roles we play. In addition to being a daughter, I work, am a mother, a wife, a friend as well as a Christian. Each of us must choose how much of our life to devote to our demented loved one. It is okay to accept help from visiting nurses, respite caregivers, friends, relatives or a nursing facility, if that is the best choice. Each of us need some balance in our life. To accept help or to place someone we love in a nursing facility is sometimes a greater act of love than to sacrifice our life for this person. No one wants to be cared for by a self-sacrificing martyr. NO ONE wants to be dependent on others. When the need arises, most people would "choose" the option of having a loving child spend regular "happy" visit times with them over the option of having a miserable, self-sacrificing person who is present all the time but not really "there."

"The person responsible for the patient's care does not also have to become a victim of the disease" (Aronson, p. 191).

EVERYONE'S SOLUTION IS NOT THE SAME

My family and my Mother and I took care of Father at home. However, we had a visiting Certified Nursing Assistant (CENA) who came three times a week to bathe him. He truly enjoyed her visits. She had a way of working with him which made him calm and accepting of care. He had a nurse who came one to three times a week depending on how sick he was. Had he lost the ability to walk, we would have had to place him in a nursing facility because we could not have done the lifting. His agility was a blessing because we were able to keep Dad home.

Is Home Care the Best Choice for YOU? (Angela Willis)

Mother felt imprisoned in my home and I could understand her frustration. I felt like the warden as well as a prisoner at the same time. The bonds that linked mother to daughter were beginning to unravel. I was so tired, so guilt ridden, so angry at myself for being so impatient with her. My husband and children were supportive as well as my siblings, but it was not enough. My brother told me to put Mom in a nursing facility, but I couldn't do it. Looking back, it was a selfish decision. I didn't put her in a nursing home for all the wrong reasons, embarrassment that I had failed her (I was a nurse, so I should have been able to care for <u>one</u> mother). What would my relatives say? Medicaid was humiliating. I felt fear and guilt over promises I could not keep.

Instead, I diminished her memory for my children by letting her last six years be seen as a painful time in their lives. Indeed, they remember some events that evoke laughter and good memories, but mostly they remember her on the floor or speaking obscenities, removing her clothing or soiling herself. They remember the pills, the wet linens, the loud TV, the night wandering. In retrospect, had I placed her in a nursing facility, the whole family could have visited any time they wished. My sisters would have seen her more often and not called to see if it was "okay." Perhaps I would have even felt less anger, less guilt for feeling so relieved that death released my bondage.

If she had been in the nursing facility at the time of her death, trained staff would have dealt with her incontinence and falls. My brothers would have felt more comfortable dropping by to see her after work, instead of trying to time visits around my family schedule.

Perhaps, I could have **enjoyed visits with her in a neutral setting.** Just perhaps, I could have remembered her joy and laughter instead of her frustration and anger. Just perhaps, I could have remained her daughter and not her jailer. Just perhaps, this story of my mother will ease the burden for someone else.

IT IS OKAY TO LET GO AND LET GOD TAKE OVER

At the end, Father's body could no longer use the food and fluids he took in. It just "went through him." On Wednesday, the nurse told us he would probably live to Saturday at most. We did not want him to die alone so we kept him at home. We did not choose hospice because we knew people with Alzheimer's disease do better if they keep the same caregivers. He got along wonderfully with his. We knew that just transporting him to the hospital could cause him great pain and may have resulted in broken bones because his bones were very brittle. We did not want him to die alone in the hospital; so we refused hospitalization. Our choice was to allow him to meet the Lord peacefully with his family by his side. He died quietly on a Thursday at 11:22 p.m. Had he been in the hospital, this would have been at the time the nurses "give report." He would have been alone. I held one hand as his breathing ceased. Mom held the other hand. He was in his own pressure-relief bed. He had two pet dogs and a pet cat with him. His grandchildren were there. This was a good death. This is the way I want to die when the time comes.

YOU NEED TO KNOW YOU DID YOUR BEST

The day Mom and Dad were beaten and robbed, they moved in with my family. They knew they could not return home, it wasn't safe, but they weren't sure they wanted to live with us either. They were accustomed to being independent—living on their own. One of my cousins was very outspoken about how I should put them in a senior citizen's apartment. In my heart I knew Dad was too much for Mom to handle alone. I knew she needed help. I talked it over with mom and dad and we agreed they would live with my family. I had to sell my home of 20-plus years and move to a home where my parents would have their own area. I told my cousin that these are MY parents and I had to be the one to decide. I told her that what she chose to do when her parents became unable to live at home alone was her business. My parents were MY family's business. A blended family can be a great blessing.

You need to know, whatever you choose to do, you have done your own personal best. Each caregiver must know their own limits. There may come a time when the promise you made to "never put your loved one in a nursing home" is no longer valid. There is a point at which the human spirit needs a rest in order to survive. There is a time when you must think past the next crisis and face some tough decisions. Although sometimes a person can be maintained at home, at other times this is not practical or safe. The difficult decision to seek resources outside the home is often painful and guilt provoking. Whether your choice is to seek respite services (temporary relief by another person or in a health care facility), assisted living, or nursing home care, you need to "forgive" yourself for making the choice. You need to know, whatever you choose to do, you have done your own personal best. There is always a well-meaning (or not as well-meaning) friend or relative who is appalled by your decisions. Pay a tribute to your loved one by saying, "I did my best and God did the rest." You are the one who must choose because you will be the one to face both the positive and negative consequences of that choice.

Open Letter to Daughters & Sons of Alzheimer Victims—Angela Willis

My mother was a wonderful, strong, very Christian woman who loved life and faced challenges with grit and wisdom. She raised children during the depression, cared for her aged and ill father, sent a son into World War II, and opened a tavern without her husband's permission or support in 1939. Her sense of Christian duty led her to open her home and heart to orphans and the homeless before most people had ever heard the word. Recovering alcoholics, the recently released mentally ill, or handicapped teens could always find a warm bed to sleep in, hot meals, and a family atmosphere in our home. My Dad just stood back and let her "do her thing." If he disagreed with her actions, we never knew it. My Dad died in my senior year of high school after a prolonged illness. Mom carried on after his death with her usual strength and drive. I thought she was invincible. She had had a heart attack when I was 12, and was diagnosed with diabetes when I was 20. She had three heart attacks within three years. She was still invincible. She beat breast cancer at 63 years of age.

I'm not sure when I first became aware of her confusion. I had noted a lot of little things, but she compensated so well that I pushed them to the back of my mind. My husband was the first to notice her memory losses. He was a police officer and was called one day to "retrieve a partially clothed woman from the riverbank." It was Mom. She said she was following the river home. Another time, she called the Sheriff's Department to report drug dealers by the river behind the house. Actually it was our kids in the swimming pool behind the house. After her getting out a couple of times, her name was put on the back of her Medic Alert necklace with our phone number. One night she was cold, so she turned the thermostat up to 110 degrees! My son came into our bedroom and his skin was burning up. I opened the bedroom door and the heat rushed up to greet me. I was terrified. I feared the furnace would blow up. After that, we put a cage over the thermostat to prevent her touching it. (She was sleeping naked in her chair with her window open.) She had not been safe around a stove for a long time, but one night she decided to fry an egg. Even with an electric stove she managed to set her sleeve on fire. My son woke up, came into my bedroom and said, "Grandma's burning." My husband and I flew out of bed in time to prevent a major disaster. Her burning sleeve had dropped onto the linoleum. The ceiling and walls were singed and some of the cupboards were damaged. After that, we never slept soundly again. I placed one-piece burner covers over each side of the stove to avoid a recurrence and installed an additional smoke alarm.

Mom fell several times too, but only had minor injuries. She fell through a glass door once during the winter months. Two teenagers saw her on the porch and dragged her back into the house. We were in the basement and hadn't realized she was up from her nap. After that, I put decals on the glass storm door so she could see it was there.

I did a lot of things wrong twenty years ago; well, not wrong, but I'd do things differently today.

Alzheimer's wasn't being diagnosed in the 70's and early 80's except on autopsy, so there was little information available to help guide us. We knew she didn't have simple dementia; her losses were much more profound and she wasn't that old. The doctor never suggested a nursing home placement. As a nurse, I thought I could handle "it" whatever "it" was. In the end "it" won. Looking back, my mother went through all the stages of Alzheimer's dementia from an inability to recognize her own children to becoming lost in a familiar neighborhood. From simple forgetfulness to profound losses of ability to dress herself, feed herself, bathe, etc. She wandered, got lost, paced, set the house on fire, became belligerent, experienced seizures, and died sitting in her chair holding her rosary beads. She told me once that she had forgotten how to pray and it scared her. She had nothing to fear. I believe God has a special place somewhere over the rainbow for those afflicted with Alzheimer's disease. Alzheimer's strips a person bare to the soul and returns them to God as children—innocent and expectant.

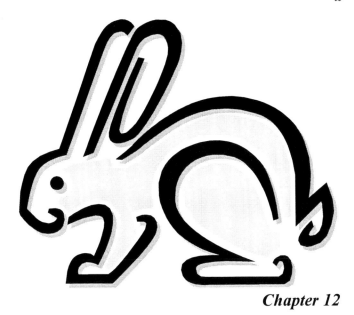

Chapter 12

DEMENTIA AND SEX

Demented people may do inappropriate things but they do not know such things are inappropriate. A demented person may take off his clothes to take a bath, forget the next step is to get into the tub and as a result, wander around naked. The nakedness is due to forgetfulness, NOT a desire to be "sexual." Father lost the ability to have sex in the beginning stage of Alzheimer's disease. A behavioral psychologist told me that this is because "sex" requires several steps and Alzheimer's dementia puts a person in the position of having to deal with life one step at a time. Research shows that the brain of a person with Alzheimer's Disease is shrunken when compared to a normal brain. This research further indicates the part of the brain which involves "judgment" is affected, meaning that while he may have known being naked was inappropriate BEFORE developing Alzheimers, he does not know it now. The dilemma is he "looks so normal" that we expect normal behavior and understanding. Possibly excluding Freud, most people would not think of a 2-year-old as a "dirty young man" when he touches his body; so why would we want to interpret the actions of an older person with a shrinking brain as those of a "dirty old man." Both the 2-year-old and the Alzheimer afflicted man "just do not know any better." Both may experience pleasure by touching their genitals but neither would know what to do after that. My experience with nakedness and dementia is that it most likely relates to something more basic, such as being hot or cold, or forgetting what to do next when taking a bath. Dad took his clothes off because he had a stone in his ureter (a tube which connects the bladder to the kidney) and was trying to make the pain stop. It wasn't until the ureter burst and he was admitted to the hospital to have it repaired, that he stopped taking his clothes off. Some Alzheimer's disease victims remove all their clothes when they need to use the bathroom. They remember "not to wet" their clothes, but the memory stops there.

One lady took her clothes off due to rectal itching, another because of hemorrhoids, a third because of a vaginal infection and itching. I have seen women rubbing their private parts in the living room in front of strangers and I've seen men who walk around holding their penis in just the same way 2-year-olds do. The point is they do not know any better. Give him or her something to hold or take him or her into the bedroom. Talk to the person and try to distract him or her. He may know it feels good but does not have the capacity to realize such behavior is socially unacceptable. Pleasure is a basic, primitive instinct. Dementia frequently takes us back to our primitive instincts.

Naomi Feil in her book The Validation Breakthrough, pp. 188-193 discusses a Dr. Willard who is a person with Alzheimer's Disease who was pinching CENAs when they try to care for him, as a man who has had brain damage and did not know how to deal with his strong emotions. She described him as releasing his strong sexual urges by pinching women. Ms. Feil used activities as well as pairing him with a female friend for activities to provide him with a socially acceptable outlet for such feelings. She explained that it was not Dr. Willard's behavior that was sexual but the Certified Nursing Assistants' interpretation of the behavior that was sexual. This has been my experience also. Virginia Morris in her book, How to Care for Aging Parents, indicates, "Inappropriate public behavior is common with dementia; inappropriate sexual behavior is not." She goes on to say, "Sometimes what is construed as sexual behavior, such as sitting outdoors naked or rubbing one's crotch, may simply be an effort to get comfortable."

Further, Dr. Peter Lichtenberg, Director, Wayne State University Gerontology Clinic indicated 10-1-98 during an interview that 95% of people with dementia lack the capacity for sex.

An interview with Beth Spencer, MSW; professor of Gerontology at Madonna University and one of the coauthors of Understanding Difficult Behavior indicated in an interview approximately 5 years ago that the majority of people who have dementia lost the ability to have sexual relations in the first stage of the disease. This is the stage when the demented person "knows" that what they think is not quite right and are constantly searching for the "truth." They cover up for their dementia and it is sometimes hard to tell whether or not they have dementia. She further indicated that she felt the reason for this loss of ability to have sex was because sexual activity requires more than one step and people with dementia can start activities but then get "lost" about what to do next. For example, one man trying to put on his shirt, slipped one arm into a sleeve and then just stood there. He couldn't remember what to do next. Had I not come along to help him, he may have just stood there for hours.

At one church owned nursing home, one demented man got in bed with another demented man. Trying to do the right thing, the Director of Nursing notified the police and Michigan authorities only to discover upon examining the situation that nothing had happened. In fact, what happened was that the Certified Nursing Assistant taking care of these men had just come to work after having worked the midnight shift at a mental facility and assumed the residents had been being sexual. When the physician was informed, he laughed and indicated that neither of the gentlemen involved had the capability of having sex due to their dementia.

I have encountered caregivers who are afraid of being "raped" by an Alzheimer patient. If such a thing were to happen, I would suggest the perpetrator may have other problems such as a psychosis and probably is not truly an Alzheimer's-afflicted person. I have also seen Alzheimer's disease as a diagnosis on someone who for some other reason was confused. A dear friend of mine had a small stroke. Because she had white hair and seemed confused, she was treated as if she had dementia. She did not. I have reviewed medical records where "Alzheimer's-type dementia" is assumed without a thorough history and mental status exam being conducted. I know that to live life fully is to take some risk. I have never worked with a demented person who did not give me more than I gave him or her. Ruth Dunkle wrote a book called DECISION-MAKING IN LONG-TERM CARE. In it she expressed a lovely sentiment which went something like, "Under that wrinkled skin, behind those confused eyes, lives a person, with feelings, emotions, thoughts—just like all of us." This person wants to be a part of life but does not know how. Please help him or her to be a part of life.

A Final Farewell to My Father

Dear Dad,

If I could say all the things I really want to say.
It might fill a dictionary, It might take all day.
I know you were still in there, even though you were confused.
I could still see "you" in your twinkling eyes and humor in there, too.

I know when you took your clothes off, you really were in pain. (kidney stones)
I know you'd never do that in a non-demented day.
I'll always remember your determination and how each hair went its way.
Your asking, "What am I supposed to do?" (Even the 400th time that day.)

I wish I would have understood better,
Before you passed away.
There is so much I know much better,
Now that you're on your way.

To share your gift of laughter,
With God and all His staff.
I'll remember you with fondness,
Especially when I laugh!

Love Debby

Chapter 13

PASTORAL

MINISTRY

SECTION*

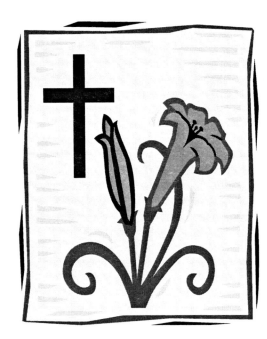 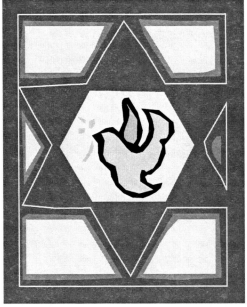

*Please note: This section is designed to stand on it's own as a separate unit. Therefore there is some information from other parts of this book which is repeated.

According to the National Interfaith Coalition on Aging, Inc. (NICA)
"Spiritual Well-Being is the affirmation of life in a relationship with God, self, community and environment that nurtures and celebrates wholeness." copyright NICA 1975.

Alzheimer's disease is a progressive deteriorating illness. It affects more than 4 million Americans (Doka, p. 119). It is marked by changes in behavior and personality and by a decline in thinking abilities. This mental decline is related to a loss of nerve cells and the links between them. Each person is different in the rate at which his or her disease progresses. The disease advances from mild forgetfulness to severe mental decline. Warning signs include, but are not limited to, loss of recent memory, impaired judgment, difficulty doing familiar tasks, problems finding the right words, disorientation to time and place, inability to do simple math, losing things, and personality changes. The person may forget how to do simple things like washing his/her hands, may no longer think clearly or remember words or family members' names (American Alzheimer Assn.).

In working with Alzheimer victims I find that when you say familiar prayers or sing familiar hymns the dementia victim can often join in singing. Sometimes the person will remember the words better than I do. I have had particular good luck with "Amazing Grace." "Emotional memories often connected with religious experiences among religious elders are among the last memories to be lost in dementing illness." (Koenig) Each person is different and should be approached from the perspective of that person's faith.

Family can be very valuable in identifying favorite hymns as well as well-loved passages from The Bible or the Tora or <u>The Book of Mormon</u> or whatever faith text is familiar to the victim. I found that as a daughter of a victim of Alzheimer's Disease that I needed to find a way to make peace of the reason why my beloved father was deteriorating in this way. When father had had colon cancer previously, I reconciled this with my faith by deciding that part of father had died and gone on to be with God before his spirit. But when he was diagnosed as having Alzheimer's I eventually accepted this as his mind going on to be with God a little at a time. In a way I thought of this as God's way of making an easier transformation for him and his loved ones when it came time to enter into the kingdom of heaven.

Problems Encountered

Ministering to the family of a person with Alzheimer's is particularly difficult. "In fact, 'because of the long-term burdens on them and the potential physical and emotional consequences, family members are recognized as the secondary victims of AD'" (Doka, pp. 119-120). As wonderful as the people who care for this person may be, they tend to repress and overlook their own needs and feelings and often do not wish to admit they have a problem, too. "Bereavement and family caregiving are treated as two separate issues but actually they are part of the same chronic situation" (Doka, p. 120). The family is faced with a number of losses. They lose their relationship with the family member affected. They lose the person they used to rely on and confide in. They lose friends and family as a result of the constant watching and caring required. In addition, the Alzheimer victim does not "look" sick and generally can walk until toward the end of the disease; so friends who have not been in this situation do not understand why the caregiver does not have time for them. Also, the caregivers do not have the time and energy to follow their personal interests on a regular basis. "Alzheimer disease has been recognized as causing the psychological death of its victims long before the actual physical death" (Doka, p. 120). As if the above losses were not enough, there is a stigma to having Alzheimer's disease because it is associated with two groups which are stigmatized—the mentally ill and the elderly. Typical family reactions tend to be the opposite of what is needed: shame, guilt, anger or embarrassment. At the time when family and friends are needed most, they are not available (Doka, p. 123-124).

Care for the Caregiver

According to <u>Caring for the Alzheimer Patient,</u> in order to have the emotional and physical strength to deal with the difficult care required, the caregiver needs to assure he or she has sufficient support, someone to confide in and plenty of time off. <u>If a minister can **get the caregiver to meet his or her own needs**, the odds are greater that nursing facility care may be delayed</u> (Dipple, p. 19). In <u>Show Me The Way To Go Home</u>, Larry Rose compares Alzheimer's disease to cancer except there is no radiation, there is no chemotherapy, there is no cure. There is just progressive deterioration to death. As the disease progresses, the importance of having a caregiver present to guide this person through the day increases. Mr. Rose describes hearing a noise and knowing it sounds familiar but not realizing it is a phone until the answering machine picks up. Mr. Rose describes getting lost in his pickup truck and having to find someone to help him. Mr. Rose is a victim of early onset Alzheimer's. But he is so intelligent (a member of Mensa which is an organization for geniuses), he is able to compensate better than the majority of victims who must give up driving much sooner than Mr. Rose. It is not uncommon for an Alzheimer victim to require step-by-step instructions just to put on a shirt. It is as though a victim can start a task but then gets stuck and does not know what to do next. One man, for example, tipped over a table. He bent down to pick it up and remained there bent over. Then 15 minutes to an hour later, when I walked by, he was still standing there bent over. I asked him what was wrong but he could not answer. I took his hands and guided them to pick up the table and place it upright. He could not talk or move or do any other task until he had worked his way through the solution for the table. After we uprighted the table, he said, "Oh, THANK YOU!" You could hear a tremendous sense of relief in his voice. Caregiving for such a person is constant, never-ending. Every time the person cannot think what to do, <u>to him</u> it can be an emergency. The person wants everything to stop and someone to come running (even if one is in the bath tub) in order for the Alzheimer victim to achieve piece of mind. This takes a terrible toll on the caregiver.

<u>The most important part of pastoral ministry to the Alzheimer victim is getting the caregiver to care for himself or herself.</u> One way of elevating caregiver spirits is to get this person to find "some magic" in each day. Magic may be watching the birds and squirrels or smelling the flowers. Magic could mean enjoying something "cute" the person had done. I know it is hard to see some of the things a demented person does as cute. However, we can get the caregiver to see the confused actions of an Alzheimer victim affectionately as those of a six-foot 2-year-old, not "bad," just confused and needing direction. Then try to get the caregiver to enjoy that part of him which is left. Both family and victim will enjoy a better quality of life. In <u>Understanding Alzheimer's Disease</u> it is suggested caregivers need to restructure their lives as well as plan for respite care on a regular basis. Further, caregivers need to be prepared for the progressive nature of the disease by being flexible. Common reactions to being informed of a progressive fatal disease include shock, anger, fear, feeling overwhelmed, loss of control, grief, guilt, anxiety, a reevaluation of beliefs, the desire to bargain, and hope (Babcock, pp. 9 - 15). A support group or someone who has been a caregiver for a person with Alzheimer's disease can be of great assistance in order to make life for both the caregiver and the victim more normal and get coping ideas. "The person responsible for the patient's care does not also have to become a victim of the disease" (Aronson, p. 191).

Closure

Unlike other types of prolonged terminal illness such as cancer, Alzheimer victims and their families do not always make arrangements for what will be done when death occurs. Often the family of the victim will be to at least some extent in denial, that is, not wanting to admit this is a fatal illness. The need to plan funeral arrangements is not identified because the victim may die within months of diagnosis or live as long as 10 years (Doka, p. 119). The illness may progress very slowly or very rapidly. My mother refused to accept the fact that father had Alzheimer's and to the day he died expected him to recover. In my father's case this actually worked to his advantage because mother would expect him to do things for himself. Because she expected it, he did it. She also would repeat instructions over and over, which again served to "empower" him to do what was asked. The down side of denial is that by the time the family realizes their loved one does have dementia, he may be too far gone for them to reach closure on unresolved feelings or issues. At that point writing about feelings and the issues in a journal or notebook or even in a letter to God in order to reach some sort of peace within one's self is a good approach. Writing in such a journal is completed when the writer thinks he or she is done. Some people write out their feelings in a journal their entire life. There is nothing wrong with this.

Family Responsibilities

Family members need to divide responsibilities. Some may require counseling in order to come up with a working arrangement all family members can agree upon. Family counseling may need to explore early family history as it relates to current family practices in order to help families also in resolution of feelings of grief, loss and guilt. The burden of caregiving becomes easier when conflicts are resolved (Dipple, p. 20-21).

One study indicated some siblings tend to get excused from caregiving based on childhood reputations as having been irresponsible or a trouble-maker as a child (Dipple. p. 20). To keep such people from the opportunity of caregiving cheats them out of the opportunity to grow. This situation sets up the "responsible" sibling to become the self-sacrificing martyr and further worsens an already-strained relationship. One study indicates the irresponsible child has greater difficulty accepting the loss of the loved one (Dipple, p. 20). It is important that a cooperative relationship exist between family members. Criticizing caregivers for what is being done is destructive and helps no one. My rule of thumb is that

unless I'm willing to assume the tasks the caregiver is assuming, I do not criticize. Praise and admiration go a long way toward elevating self-esteem and lifting the burden a bit for caregivers. **Complimenting the caregiver for a job well done and telling them how difficult it is** can help to lift the burden a bit. Such compliments can help caregivers recharge and keep on going.

Honor Thy Father and Mother

Even though what my father was saying or doing may not have made sense, he was still my father and I treated him with respect. I always made a point to make eye contact with him and treat issues he saw as serious, seriously. He would say things like, "What am I going to do about Uncle Will's house?" Now I may know Uncle Will passed on before I was born, but I would say, "What do you think we should do, Dad?" He would then say, "They're going to sell it to perfect strangers." Then I would say, "What do you think we should do." He would reply, "I guess there's not much we can do." Mother was with father 24 hours a day. Father slept very little. There were times when she did not make much sense due to sleep deprivation. Sometimes I would need to take off work to drive them somewhere if I knew she was too tired. If she were insistent we do something a specific way, then I would honor her request as best I could. There were times when she would want to tell me off and yell and scream at me because I was there. I would find something to do in a distant part of the house until she calmed down. It was not me she was yelling at, it was the Alzheimer's disease whose existence she refused to acknowledge.

Permission to Have Feelings

One of the greatest gifts one can give an Alzheimer victim or his family is permission to feel the way this person feels. I have yet to meet a caregiver who did not lose his or her temper and yell in anger at the victim at one time or another. This is almost always accompanied by extreme guilt and embarrassment in addition to self-condemnation. It is okay to get angry sometimes. I tell caregivers one of the benefits of losing one's temper with an Alzheimer victim is he won't remember it. Family members need to use different ways of venting in order to avoid being injured, however. We need to try to avoid yelling and arguing with the victim because this tends to cause combative behavior by the victim. People are human and humans lose their temper once in a while. Hitting the victim is not an acceptable way to respond.

An ounce of prevention is worth a pound of cure: It is not unusual for Alzheimer victims to repeat the same acts over and over. There is such a strength of will to this repetitive activity. If possible, it should be permitted, unless injury or harm may result. One effective way we can reduce anxiety for caregivers is to remove from the person's area of influence any dangerous substances or sharp objects. The victim's perception of objects is skewed. He may think he is handing you a fly swatter when he is actually handing you a knife by the sharp end. I follow the rule that I do not leave within the victim's reach objects or chemicals I would not allow a 2-year-old child to have. When Dad was in an agitated state, we locked doors in rooms we did not want him in; he could still walk around but had less opportunity to hit his head. Once Dad had a severe urinary tract infection and wasn't making much sense. He would not stay in bed and every time he got up, he fell. After he had fallen three times in 15 minutes, I decided enough was enough. Instead of arguing with him over staying in bed, I just told him to stay on the floor. Dad laid on the floor with a pillow and blanket for a while and then he did better when he got up. My reasoning behind this solution was he was going to hurt himself, and encouraging him to stay on the floor prevented injury. You can't fall up! These are just some suggestions. There are no absolute quick-fixes a person can do to remedy everything. The same solution does not always work, even if the problem **looks** the same. That is why the Behavior Tracking Form is useful. I use it to keep a list of what works and what has worked. That way, even though an approach may not be working now, it may work in the future. One good idea for preventing problem behavior, though, is to look to see if one can tell what the person is reacting to; that is, what was this person doing directly before the behavior began—or what happened which set him going? If you can remove the stimulus which is causing the behavior, often the behavior will stop or not occur. For example, some victims scream when taking a shower because their sense of touch has also been affected by the disease. Why not have him take a bath instead? Why should everyone endure screaming, if it is preventable?

Caregiver Health Problems: There is no more difficult role than the role of the caregiver. No one should sacrifice himself or herself by constantly caring for a demented person without help or respite. Caring for a person with Alzheimer's drains caregivers physically, emotionally and spiritually. Caregivers are often elderly and this, combined with the fact that Alzheimer victims tend not to sleep at night, provides additional stress. At the very least caregivers need to plan respite help and/or accept help. "[O]ne common predictor of nursing facility placement is the primary caregiver's physical disability as the patient care demands increase" (Doka, p. 125). One of the pastoral ministry challenges in this situation is convincing the family when placement in a supervised care setting or nursing facility is what is best for the victim. No one wants to put mom or dad in a nursing facility, but the pastoral minister can best assist both the victim and the family by getting them to accept the reality of the care needed. Ask the family what they would want if they were the ones who had Alzheimer's Disease. The most tragic thing I have seen is a son who died of a heart attack trying to do everything himself taking care of his mom who did not recognize him. She then went on to live in a nursing facility where she is fine. If he had taken her to the nursing facility when the burden became too great or accepted help such as respite caregivers, I wonder if he might not still be alive. **Solution-Focus:** Solution-focused therapy (Goldberg, p. 308) presents a good example of ministering methods which may be used to help the victims cope with the devastating effects of the progressive degeneration of Alzheimer's disease. Rather than dwelling on the unfairness of the disease or their situation, **support should be focused on what can be done to improve the situation and quality of life of all involved.** Life may not seem fair sometimes, but **God is good.** We need to look for solutions which will work for "this" family, solutions which they can accept and carry out. The focus is on problem solving and defining the time to make a change. It is important to encourage caregivers to accept help, take time for themselves and release resentments over their life journey. Probably the most important support we can give the family is to get them to establish contacts with a support group or other families which have experienced what they are now going through. Ministers need to encourage coping strategies which may include journal writing, listening to music, working through grief, fear, anger, and crisis in faith. Families need to work their way through each day with as much joy as possible. They need to know the mom or dad they've loved all these years is still there but can no longer access all of his or her memories and has difficulty with judgment. We need to help families find new ways to cope. We need to turn our cares over to the Heavenly Father and allow him to care for us.

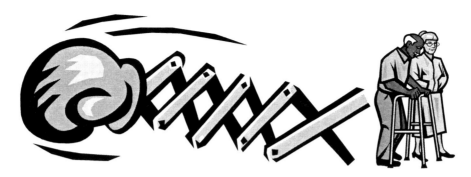

HOW NOT TO GET HIT WHEN MINISTERING TO PEOPLE WHO HAVE THE "LABEL" DEMENTIA

1. Make **eye contact**, <u>wear a pleasant expression</u> on your face. A simple **"hello"** spoken with affection can mean more than volumes of conversation or unwanted reading from scripture. The person may not be able to understand scripture anymore. But, human contact is so important to these modern day untouchables.

2. **Keep conversation simple**, use simple words, see how the person reacts, then try to speak to her at her level of understanding. A Children's Bible might come in handy also.

DO NOT "TALK ***DOWN***" TO THE PERSON. She STILL has feelings which can be hurt. If the person does not appear to be understanding your words, then 2 possible causes can be:

    a. **Hard of hearing**? Try using words on paper - or pointing - touch her gently to provide reassurance.

    b. Dementia may be related to clogged arteries in the brain (multi-infarct dementia is one label). <u>Only part of what you are saying may be heard:</u>
        i) **speak louder and clearer**
        ii) **use simple words**
        iii) **use 4 word sentences** such as "follow me, this way" rather than "if you will follow me, we will go to the main dining room." (too many words to understand)

    c. **Repeat your 4 word sentence several times** as each time that person may get a little more of the message. It is like plugged plumbing. If you try to pour a bucket of water down a stopped sink fast, you will end up spilling water over the edge of the sink. But if you pour water a little at a time, eventually it will all go down the drain.

3. **Try not to startle the person**, or grab her. Try not to put the person in a situation with too much noise or where there is too much background activity or noise. <u>The more noise and activity there is, the more the demented person's ability to understand will diminish.</u>

4. **Change the subject.** If this person continues to "focus" her thoughts on one concept (such as "My mother needs me home to do the dishes."), ask about her mother **or try to repeat what she is saying;** then change the subject. "Oh, your mother needs you home to do the dishes. You must be a good daughter; what is your mother like?"

5. <u>DO NOT ARGUE WITH THIS PERSON</u>. There is no better way to get hit than to argue. She needs to know you accept her as she is.

6. **Do not try to "force" the person to do something. Instead suggest 1 or 2 alternatives** and ask which she would like. (*DO NOT OFFER AN ALTERNATIVE WHICH WOULD ENCOURAGE HER TO DO WHAT SHE IS ATTEMPTING TO DO WHICH IS NOT OKAY.*) For example, "I want to go home, right now." Say, "Oh you want to go home right now, but I

came to visit you. Should we go to the dining room or the day room?" Or ask her to tell you about "home" AND why she wants to go there.

7. Remember, this person is a child of God, your brother or sister under Christ. **When a person has dementia, being treated with respect and dignity becomes increasingly important.** Respect can allow someone with Alzheimer's dementia to do more than she reasonably should be able to do, because it is expected of her.

WHAT IF THE PERSON DOES BECOME COMBATIVE?

<u>Try not to put yourself in a situation where you are 'cornered.'</u> I had a 6-foot 5-inch very strong demented person corner me in a room. He then began to come after my throat with his hands. There was no door or window except behind him. One of the things a person loses when they get dementia is his or her inhibitions relating to inappropriate behavior. This person is not necessarily mentally ill. I just think of it as though his brain were a switchboard with some of the wires connected wrong.

Look to see what he or she was doing directly before becoming difficult and try to avoid that happening again.

For example, once when Mom and I took Dad out to eat at a restaurant, he looked at the menu and started swearing and took a swing at my Mom. What was the trigger for the behavior? The menu—too many hard choices, too complicated. **His anger was a reaction to the frustration of not being able to figure out what to do.**

After that, we learned to:

1) Not give him a menu.
2) Not argue with him.
3) Offer him two choices.

He would say, "What do I want to eat?" To which we would reply, "Today you're in the mood for meatloaf and coffee." He would then say, "That sounds good."

Chapter 14

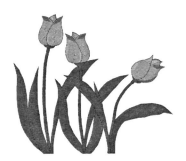

Ladies' Discussion Group

As a part of Mrs. Bastedo's Mental Health Specialist training, she did a study of demented women living in a nursing facility setting and how they interacted in a ladies' group discussion. Although it really was a dementia victims' group, we called it the "Ladies' Discussion Group." The original idea was loosely patterned after another study done with people with early dementia. The study referenced was done by the Early Stage Alzheimer's Program in the Greater Houston Chapter of the Alzheimer's Association in 1993. (Reichlin, 168)

The dementia victims from their study were chosen from an adult day care situation and were living with their family in the community. This group also had family group support meetings in order to help the families understand, cope with and reinforce the goals of their study. In addition the people's strengths were identified so the families could see them. The Houston Group were higher functioning without the severity of illness of the Ladies' Discussion Group. For this study they developed specific criteria for acceptance into their group. They indicated that in order to participate, a person must have intact social and communication skills, have similar educational backgrounds and life experiences. The people selected were recommended by staff. In the selected group, five people met twice a week. The group leaders suggested particular themes to generate discussion. The meetings were videotaped and discussed by the group at the following meeting. (Reichlin, 168).

Ladies' Discussion Group criteria for acceptance:

- Must be a woman
- Must be able to speak more than just a couple of words or repeating a phrase.
- Must not have severe medical conditions like open wounds, tube feeding, oxygen, or be bedridden.
- Must be able to sit upright.
- Must be able to make eye contact
- Must be able to sit in a room for 45 minutes
- Must be capable of being socially acceptable during the group meeting.

In the Ladies Discussion Group it was necessary to modify the format used by the Houston study in order to accommodate the ladies with whom I was working. Our hypothesis was that if we were to put higher functioning ladies with more impaired ladies, the more impaired ladies might do better and perhaps participate more. We had residents with differing abilities and differing levels of dementia. We chose ladies in order to avoid the confounding factors presented when men and women are together.

OUR LADIES

We attempted to take the best qualities of the study as noted above and generalize them to a long term care setting. We got permission slips from family members in order to video tape the ladies who attended. We wanted to do 6 sessions one week apart but ended up doing 5 sessions which were not done one after the other. There were always two people working with the group, myself and another staff member for safety reasons. We wanted to accept as group members ladies who were not all the same in terms of culture mental status or background. Our theory was that the more capable ladies would assist the more severely impaired ladies to interact. We wanted to know the mental status of the ladies as well as check each for depression before proceeding. We did the Mini Mental State Exam and began by doing the Geriatric Depression Scale. This scale, as well as, the Mini Mental Examination were indicated as valid in comprehensive geriatric assessment. (Boult, 2001, 3.) Two of the ladies who participated were mildly impaired, four ladies were moderately impaired and four ladies were severely impaired. In the beginning, we used the Geriatric Depression Scale but had to discontinue it because ladies would drop out after taking it. This instrument contains questions one asks the person being assessed but the questions seemed to make the ladies feel depressed. One lady was so upset after answering the questions that she had her daughter call and rescind permission to attend. So instead we used the Cornell Scale for Depression in Dementia, which is based on subjective observation by the person doing it. Using this scale, we had only one person who tested as depressed and she left after attending only part of one group. We started out with 40 potential group members but narrowed that down to 10 women who actually participated. We had ladies from 71 to 97 years of age with the average age being 87. None of the ladies came to every session. We usually had 4 ladies at each group, 3 during one session. We did insist that the ladies who participated have the ability to talk.

We wanted to empower the women so we had the women chose what they wanted to discuss. While we did try some of the exercises from the previous study, our ladies just wanted to talk. Our focus became empowerment and attempting to help these demented ladies feel "normal." Our one rule was, "It is okay not to be able to remember things, we all do it sometimes." If a lady wanted to leave, we let her leave. We asked each of the ladies if they wanted to come before each meeting and if they said no, it meant no. While our ladies said they did not remember having been in the ladies discussion group, their facial expression changed when they saw us after attending the group and their participation became better and more active as the meetings progressed. The group leaders introduced each of the ladies who then each told a little about themselves. It did not matter what they told us, it was up to them.

During our first meeting, the ladies sat expressionless and waited for us to tell them what to do. We continued to go around the circle of ladies asking them their opinions or what they would like to talk about. Every lady participated. One lady (May) had a severe physical impairment and a neurological disease. But she participated too. She was very weak. During our first meeting the ladies discussed where they each had grown up and their religion briefly. Toward the end of this meeting May's face lit up and she said, "Good, Fun!"

One lady (Jane) who tested severely impaired was very quiet and would even sleep during the meetings. But we kept encouraging her to make choices and by the last session, she was smiling ear to ear and talking our arms off. Jane had multi-infarct dementia. Sometimes what she said sounded like gibberish to us but if you looked at what she might be saying, and made a guess, she would find it so comforting to be heard. She was talking away and when she finished I said, "It is very frustrating to be trying to say something and not be able to get the words to come out." She said, "yes." Her sister Amy would boss Jane around and Jane would follow her around all day. But Jane would get angry about this and take off sometimes. Telling her it was okay not to remember was very empowering for her. Amy is almost deaf. Jane can read but Amy cannot. Amy tested as moderately impaired while Jane tested as severely impaired. By the end of our meetings, Jane had established her independence from Amy and no longer followed Amy around. At first this was distressing to Amy but eventually she found someone else in a wheelchair and she was okay. Amy was very anxious, especially if she could not remember something. She enjoys conversation but has difficulty getting facts straight. Amy had experienced encepalopathy and her brain had been without oxygen for a time. She became very upset when she spilled a glass of water. Amy is distressed sometimes because she cannot remember her history and sometimes does not remember she has a daughter.

Joy was born in Montreal and tested as mildly impaired. She loves to talk and enjoyed group very much. After attending several sessions, she would just show up in the office on the day and at the time we were having meetings. When I asked her if she was coming to our Ladies' Discussion Group, she would say she didn't know what that was and said she didn't remember it. But then she said, "What are we going to talk about? Are you going to take our pictures today?" One of the other ladies asked Joy if she was a man because her hair was cut short. So for the last meeting she put on rouge and lipstick and eyebrow pencil.

Haley tested as mildly impaired. She still makes life choices and runs her own affairs. She signed her own permission slip. Haley was the life of the party when she attended. She joked and was cheerful and asked the other women to "tell me about your boyfriends" While she does not know factual information, she loved to talk to the other ladies.

Thelma speaks rapidly in what sounds like gibberish because the words are not always related. But when we listened to her, she would slow down and she was able to get three or four words in a row correct. She has difficulty hearing and extremely bad eyesight. She speaks Polish. She has a limited fund of information, knows her first name but not her last. She truly enjoyed our group and loved being listened to.

Heidi is a 93 year-old widow. She tested as moderately impaired. She has a pancreatic tumor and respiratory difficulty which complicate her dementia. She really enjoyed group and loved to talk about growing up in Germany. She told us how hungry she had been during the World War and after our meeting had 3 sandwiches in a row. Heidi was a very willing participant.

Emily was our youngest participant at 71 years of age but also our most depressed. She is the only lady who scored as having depression. She expressed fears that the other ladies were talking about her. She was only able to attend part of one meeting because she became hysterical and asked to leave. Emily's hysterics definitely sounded like a fear response. She obsesses over wanting to die. She tested as moderately impaired. Psychologists Jerome and Julia Frank would possibly say that because Esther loathes herself, it is possible that she feared and disliked the other ladies in the group because she perceives them as like herself and expected they would loathe her too. (Frank and Frank, 1991)

Daisy tested as moderately impaired on the Mini Mental State Exam. Daisy has a short attention span and found it difficult to join in appropriately. She also has poor short-term memory. She tends to respond by repeating the same sentence over and over and does not say many other words.

Betty tested as severely impaired. She is on Haldol (an antipsychotic medication). She enjoyed telling us about what it was like to come to America from Poland. She speaks Polish but has trouble with some words in Polish. She is hard of hearing. She uses a wheelchair. As I wheeled her from group, she said, "Thank you so much for inviting me, I felt like I was home."

WHAT THE LADIES LIKED:

They liked to talk about where they grew up. Haley asked everyone to tell about their boyfriends. Amy told us what it was like to grow up in Hamtramck, Michigan. Heidi told us what it was like to grow up in Germany. They also enjoyed talking about their different religions. They liked being asked their opinion about everything we did. They liked being treated as equals by the coleaders who do not have dementia. They liked having the freedom to choose and learn about other women who live where they live. They liked socializing as adults in a group of peers.

NOTICEABLE CHANGES IN BEHAVIOR

At first everyone was nervous but after a little coaching participated freely. Even though some of our ladies were fairly cognitively impaired, they managed to participate each in her own way. Our Ladies' Discussion Group provided our ladies with an opportunity to make choices and direct their own activity. This was very empowering for them. Just because someone is impaired and does not know who the president is doesn't mean they do not like to talk. After the first group meeting, when I saw the ladies in the hall, they appeared more confident and more talkative than before group. Joy liked to crack jokes and was very empowered. Actually except for Emily and Daisy who would not stay for the meeting, all the ladies showed signs of empowerment as evidenced by their smiles, gestures, body language, and what they said.

WHAT I LEARNED

- Assessment forms appropriate for geriatric people may not be appropriate for demented geriatric people.
- Mixing mild to severe dementia victims in a nursing facility setting does facilitate discussion and does stimulate both the moderate and the severe stage dementias, provided their personalities are compatible with group activity.
- Some demented people cannot go to group meetings, especially if they are unable to converse or they are severely emotionally impaired.
- In a nursing facility or other setting where the people are very sick with severe medical conditions and multiple problems, it is wise to have a pool of participants from whom to choose for meetings.
- Many of the ladies were assessed toward the end of our project. That gave me the advantage of not knowing how impaired they would test. Therefore, we treated them all alike.
- I learned that the degree of impairment does not have a lot to do with a person's ability to socialize and join social settings.
- The more patient we were, the better the ladies became at participating.

A NEW STUDY

In "THE NUN STUDY," Steve Liss studied 678 nuns to understand what encourages a person to maintain maximum ability in mental function. Steve Liss indicated "stimulating the brain with continuous intellectual activity keeps neurons healthy and alive." (Lemonick & Mankato, 2001, 62) Logically it follows that the discussion of information in a group might prove stimulating also, even in someone who is already impaired. The Alzheimer Care Center in Chicago has found that for some people with dementia, talking to peers can offer them solace. (Kalb, 2000, 53). Dr David Bennett, director of the Alzheimer's Disease Center at Chicago's Rush-Presbyterian-St. Luke's Medical Center, said, "Even though they can't do what they used to do, that doesn't mean they can't enjoy life at the moment," (Kalb, 52) In one study, simple conversation about favorite foods or whatever, "helped reduce by half the disruptive verbal outbursts of nursing home residents with dementia." (Kalb, 54) It would appear possible that by being in the Ladies' Discussion Group, the participants' desire to socialize might be increased as evidenced by the increased social contact observed in the participants after being group members. "Mastering the complex social demands of the setting (patients who are confused in any treatment setting) helps rebuild patients' sense of self-efficacy and competence." (Frank & Frank, 1991, 286)

Our hypothesis that treating dementia victims the way you would treat anyone else would improve their ability to function proved correct. Being in a mixed group of mildly, moderately, and severely impaired victims proved to be empowering for them all. The right to refuse is a very powerful thing for any person living in an institutional setting. It is especially powerful for dementia victims. By virtue of their disease symptoms and confusion, they are often forced to do things they do not want to do, nor do they understand why such things are necessary. The reward of seeing how much people who have dementia perk up when they are allowed to take charge and choose is well worth the amount of waiting required to allow them the time to choose. Observation suggests that participation in a group with peers is confidence building, provides solace, and gives the participants a sense of mastery and encourages them to try socializing in other settings.

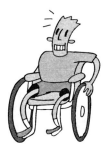

Chapter 15

ASSESSING

What is the first step?

AT HOME:

FIRST STEP: The first step in deciding what to do for a victim of dementia is to look to see what is NOT causing the behavior. This would be a good time to have a physician or nurse practitioner do a check up on this person to make sure there are no physical problems which may be causing this behavior. For example, urinary tract infections, lung problems, heart problems, infection of any kind, hemorrhoids, constipation, being dehydrated. This is especially true if the behavior came on suddenly rather than gradually over time. If the reason for the behavior is medical, trying to avoid repeat behavior will not be as effective because this type of cause for a problem needs to be treated first in order to reveal the real dementia process.

SECOND: Use the reminder list, "Factors to Check for Prior to Behavioral Management" located in this book. Keep a list of conditions which made the person's behavior worse previously on the behavior tracking record. Such as, he became aggressive when he had a urinary tract infection. Watch the person's body language to see where he appears to be hurting. See the section on pain for further information on this subject.

THIRD: Communicate with your nurse practitioner or physician. See the form which is entitled, "Behavior Recommendations." The idea is to provide the nurse or practitioner with your insight as to what has been happening with your loved one. You are with this person every day, you see what he or she does.

FOURTH: Once we have looked and cannot find any medical reason for the behavior, then we begin watching this person. What happens directly before the behavior occurs? Is it when things are too noisy? Is it because someone moved a favorite piece of furniture? Is it because someone is arguing with this person? Does it occur when you try to keep the person from doing something he/she wants to do? Does it happen when the person changes his clothing or takes a shower?

FIFTH: Once you decide what you think is causing the problem, you look for a solution which removes what occurs which causes this person to act the way he or she acted. For example, if noisy environments are upsetting then move the person away from the noise. If it is because someone argues with the person then explain to that person that arguing upsets him/her and causes this person to become distressed. Sometimes you literally need to ask the arguing person to either leave or stop arguing. Agree the arguer is correct, but that they are causing problems. It is not important whether something a demented person believes is right or wrong. Perhaps this is the only thing the demented person knows is true about his world. Demented people most generally lose the ability to understand what is socially correct. They act on what they think they need. If it is not moving furniture, do not move furniture unless the dementia victim is not present. If you must keep the person from doing something. Try distraction or diplomacy. One lady tried repeatedly to get on the elevator but was not allowed to get on the elevator. Had the caregiver argued with her, she would have become combative (someone tried this approach.) But instead offer her your hand and tell her there is someone who would like to speak to her or ask her if she will help you with something. Then give her something to do. If the behavior occurs when you are assisting her with dressing then it is possible that the way she is being dressed is painful for her. Try to get her to help as much as you can or try a different approach. Allowing her to help will make the activity less scary.

LASTLY: People change as well as the reasons behind the distressing behavior change. Caregivers need to constantly watch out for clues as to why this person acts in this way. Sometimes we need to vary solutions as the same solution may not always work. It is better if we have several ideas about what we can try. This is the advantage of planning.

Once we eliminate conditions which cause the dementia to worsen, then our approaches to the pure behavior become much more effective. There is a book entitled <u>Understanding Difficult Behavior</u> in the bibliography. It is a good reference for ideas on what to try for different difficult behaviors. Each person is unique and does dementia in his or her own way. Therefore as dementia caregivers we need to discover this person's way of being demented, so we can change the cause to stop the behavior and increase the quality of life for both victim and caregiver.

IN THE NURSING FACILITY SETTING:

Mrs. Bastedo was called in to assist a nursing facility because this facility was in danger of losing their license to operate. The problem which they had been unable to solve was that 80% of the nursing facility population were on antipsychotic medications without written reasons justifying the use of such drugs. Doctors and psychiatrists and behavior specialists had already come in and tried to correct the problem, but still the facility was unable to pass the requirements as reviewed by surveyors from the state of Michigan. Administration had set up a multidisciplinary team of social services, therapists, activities, dietary and nursing which were working together. However, they had not been able to conquer the requirements for use of antipsychotic drugs. The psychiatrists would change the drugs each person was receiving but did not evaluate what could be causing the behavior or environment or complicating problems such as infections or pneumonia. One resident had been given antipsychotic medication for pneumonia. What she really needed was antibiotics. But the confused behavior from pneumonia symptoms "looked" like dementia. Changing the medications alone often caused much unrest and increased symptoms for many people. Prior to observing each person, I followed the below-listed process in order to screen out complicating conditions.

First, I reviewed the medical records to see what reasons each person may have to be acting out. At the above noted facility the physicians discontinued ALL antipsychotic drugs, for all residents on this type of medication, except those for residents with a long-term mental illness history. This helped greatly because these kind of medications sometimes cover up the real reason for the behavior. Because at the time there were almost no available medications which were designed for use with dementia victims, antipsychotic medications were the medications the physicians had been using. At the end of this chapter is a reminder list for "When is it okay to ask the physician for antipsychotic medications?" We learned from this experience that the answer to this question is ONLY AS A LAST RESORT!

Second, I developed a reminder list of SOME of the factors to consider and verify before beginning a behavior management plan. Obviously there are other factors, but this list helped me to remember some of the many problems which "look" like dementia but are not dementia.

Third, I developed a communication form in order to be able to communicate important information I had found and to request specific lab work from the physician. The attending physician helped considerably in this way.

Fourth, once I had ruled out complicating issues, **I met with staff members as well as residents to gain staff insight** as well as see first hand what might be causing the residents to act inappropriately. If a Certified Nurse's Assistant is especially good working with a resident with behavior problems, ask this person what type of things he or she finds effective in working with the demented person.

Using what we learned, we developed the behavior management care plan. This was the hardest task because state surveyors kept rejecting the words being used on the patient care plan which is required. Ultimately, I took one of their citations which specifically listed the behavior, as well as the factors which triggered the behavior, the interventions which worked and those which did not work. Using the surveyor's words, I developed the care plan with the name "Mary Martin" in the care plan section. I faxed this care plan (which I had written directly from the citations) to the surveyor, who indicated this care plan was fine. Using this one care plan as an example, I went on to create care plans of this nature for other residents. The other care plan samples in the last section of this book are from other facilities in order to give you care plans not only on people from the facility who had been medicated but also other facilities.

Lastly we recognized that people change, and the reasons underlying behavior change. Caregivers are never really done checking and rechecking. We may find there would be a new cause for a behavior, or a new behavior. A specific intervention may no longer work. The book entitled Understanding Difficult Behavior (see Bibliography) offers many different ideas for behavior management. I have found it to have many simple and effective ways to manage behavior. Please see the bibliography for more information about this wonderful book.

We have discussed many conditions which can cause sudden changes in behavior as well as mimic dementia symptoms. The major reason to spend time making certain such conditions do not exist is to reveal the underlying **real behavior** for this person. Once conditions which cause dementia-like symptoms or worsen already existing dementia are eliminated, we can be much more effective in ANY technique we use to help a demented person because we will have eliminated problems which can make behavior unmanageable. The most important thing to remember is that each person does dementia in his or her own way. Therefore, caregivers have to respond in a way which **works for this person.**

FACTORS TO CHECK FOR PRIOR TO BEHAVIOR MANAGEMENT

Name: _____ Room: _____ Prior living: _____

Pertinent Social History: _____

_____ Age: _____

Diagnosis: _____

____Impaired Speech ____Difficulty Understanding ___HOH ___Vision Problem

Observed Behavior: _____

_____

_____

_____

How long has the behavior been occurring?

_____

Does behavior occur _____ BEFORE eating _____AFTER eating _____Shift Change

Medications which may affect behavior?_____

_____

Abnormal Lab: _____

_____

Cardiovascular: _____

_____

Respiratory:_____

_____

Urinary Tract Problems: _____

_____

Pain Evidence: _____

_____

Hydration: _____

_____

Weight Loss/Gain: _____

Potential Delirium Indicators: _____

_____

What have we tried? _____

ACTION Plan:_____

_____

_____

_____

FACTORS TO CHECK FOR PRIOR TO BEHAVIOR MANAGEMENT
Line by Line Suggestions on how to complete this form

Name: _____ **Room:** _____

Prior living: Write the most recent living arrangement whether alone or with son or daughter or in a nursing facility, etc.

Pertinent Social History: In this category indicate whether married and who is the person's family, where this person worked, if he or she worked; the shift they worked is good to know especially if this person worked midnights or afternoons. Indicate factors such as isolation or possible environmental contamination. Had this person always been a loner. For example, one couple on an Island in a rather isolated area. Such isolation can be a factor but the fact that both husband and wife became confused at the same time suggested possible environmental factors such as water purity.

Age: While I note age, it does not generally affect which approach I use in terms of what to do about it. Age and amount of confusion are not related.

Diagnosis: Specific information about the kind of dementia can be very useful. Often this is not available but CT scans can be very useful and also EEGs in terms of specifically describing the problems detected. Metabolic diseases such as diabetes, hypothyroidism, etc. also can have an effect on mental clarity. All current active diagnoses should be considered in terms of the effect they have on a person's ability to think.

Impaired Speech and Difficulty Understanding This is especially a problem with people who have multiinfarct dementia. They talk to you in gibberish but they are not nuts. They have lost their ability to speak clearly. Often, they know what they want to say but cannot say it. They tend to express relief and slow down when I say, "You know what you want to say but it won't come out." Sometimes they will say, "Oh, yes.!"

HOH Being hard of hearing is embarrassing. So often people will try to answer what they think you are saying. If they are incorrect they sound demented. But once we know they cannot hear we can communicate better with them and they will make more sense. I worked with one lady on 3 different days. It wasn't until the third day that I realized she wasn't demented, she was deaf.

Vision Problems: These sense categories can be very useful. Often I find hard of hearing people will be treated as demented because they cannot hear what people are saying. One lady would talk to the nurses station. The psychiatrist wrote that she was delusional. But when I watched her I noticed that the things she was saying made sense. She was just about blind and she knew the nurses were behind the station. So asking questions like, "where am I supposed to go?" Makes sense when considering she could not see very well.

Observed Behavior: It is important to notice what happens right before the behavior begins. Body language is important. Confused people will often do the "pee pee" dance very much like toddlers. Sometimes they know they need to do something but cannot remember what.

How long has the behavior been occurring? It is important to notice how often a behavior is occurring. This helps us to understand if the person's behavior is happening more often. If we know that on June 5th this person began new medication, and his behavior began to get worse on June 7th then we need to know the medication side effects and/or ask the person's doctor to review for a different medication if possible. Sometimes there is nothing that can be done.

One physician admitted he knew the cardiac medication was making this person more confused but without this medication, the person would die. The physician felt the cardiac medication was the best choice for this person.

When any person takes a sedative, hypnotic, psychotropic or other medication known for making a person feel foggy there tends to be a lessening of ability to understand the world around us. But if a demented person takes such a medication, it tends to make an already confusing world more confusing. Often this is seen when the person becomes upset and screams or tries to escape this feeling. Sometimes a demented person will strike out at other people because he or she does not know who they are and is afraid this unknown person will harm them.

Does behavior occur ___BEFORE eating ___AFTER eating __Shift Change: When reviewing behavior, one needs to know if there is a pattern to the problem. One man would get really agitated between 2:30 and 4 in the afternoon. Being diabetic, his blood sugar would be low then. We learned that if we gave him a snack at 2:00 p.m., he stopped yelling at everyone.

Another man would get up and fall every day at 2:30 in the morning. It turns out that he worked the midnight shift all his life and this was his time to eat lunch and go to the bathroom and talk to others. We learned that if we toileted him and give him a sandwich, he would go back to bed and sleep the entire night.

Medications which may affect behavior? One person I assessed had about 12 different medications. Because he was on so many medications, the odds were good the medications might be affecting him. A drug book said that the medications which he was taking interact together. I also look for side effects. The most telling fact about which medication is affecting the person is to see which medication was begun, increased or decreased close to the time the behavior began.

One lady became agitated because a bossy lady kept telling her what to do. She began throwing china vases. The physician assumed that she was not receiving enough antipsychotropic medication and he increased the medication she was taking and added an antianxiety medication as well as a medication to make her sleep. Before he increased her medications in this way she was having 12-14 behavior problems a month. After he increased her medications she began having 12-14 behavior problems every 2 weeks. Her behavior problems had doubled. It turns out that what she really needed was for the bossy lady to leave her alone.

Abnormal Lab: I consider all abnormal reports. The most frequently noted cause of behavior problems I have seen would probably be symptomless urinary tract infections. For example, one man had been living on a dementia unit for two years. Then during a routine physical, a urinalysis was done. It indicated a urinary tract infection. The physician treated it and the man stopped being confused and was able to go home. It was like a miracle. Usually, though, the improvement is not so dramatic. Having a urinary tract infection often complicates confusion. But once treated, the person becomes better but not cured of dementia.

Fasting blood sugar which is constantly low or high can cause confusion. Elevated white blood cells can be evidence of infection. A BUN of 23 or above can be an indication that more fluid intake is needed. We need to go with caution on this though because sometimes if someone has a kidney problem or pulmonary problem additional fluids can be bad for them. A physician needs to evaluate.

A low thyroid level can indicate too much thyroid is being given. Electrolyte imbalance can keep a person from using fluids or food taken in. Abnormal lab levels can be looked up and referred to the physician for help in resolving them if possible.

Cardiovascular: Write down any diagnoses which are cardiovascular in order to know in what way circulation is impaired. Sometimes there will be blood vessels which are clogged and this makes the person more demented.

Respiratory: Write down any respiratory problems. According to the clinical guidelines for care of the elderly published by the United States, when oxygen is not received adequately because of respiratory conditions, the person will be more confused. Sometimes people become combative and disoriented as a result of pneumonia.

Urinary Problems: Frequently symptomless urinary tract infections, dribbling of urine, lack of ability to clean oneself properly, etc. can lead to infection. Because demented people are confused, often they do not clean themselves properly after going to the toilet. The result is often a urinary tract infection. Because often this problem in the elderly does not have symptoms or the confused person cannot tell you he or she hurts. The only symptom may be the agitated behavior.

Pain Evidence: Look for wiggling, grimace, striking out at others when approached, verbal expressions of pain such as, "it hurts, it hurts," sliding out of the chair (especially for people with spinal degeneration), curling up, drawing one's legs into a fetal position, hitting ones arms or legs against walls or furniture, especially if the same extremity is hit over and over. One woman kept hitting her right arm against everything. When x-rayed, the arm indicated osteopenic degeneration of the bone. This was her way of telling us her arm hurt. If you asked her she would say no, it doesn't hurt but if you watch what she did you realized that it did hurt. Her arm hurt so she hit it against things to make the hurt stop. When father had pain under his colostomy, he would punch his abdomen. Please see chapter on pain.

Hydration: Look for furrowed tongue, thin fragile skin, frequent skin tears. Also, look at nutrition when skin tears begin "appearing." If this person's BUN lab work is 23 or above then probably more water is needed unless renal disease or other restriction is present. Check with the dietitian or physician as to whether more water would benefit this person. Indicators of more fluid need include but are not limited to: urinary tract infection, pneumonia or infection anywhere, skin tears, paled dehydrated look-sunken eyes, skin sunken in, pressure ulcers, on stool softeners, constipation, on pain medication or antidepressant medication.

Weight Loss: Watch for not just dramatic loss of 7 or more pounds in a week (possible dehydration), but also for a gradual unplanned weight loss of 1-2 pounds over months. It is important to pay attention to weight history and what is normal for this person. My daughter, for example, has always been under the ideal weight range for her height from the time she was a baby. For someone like her, being low weight is normal. So it is important to know what she usually weighs in order to know whether her weight is really low or if low weight is normal for the person.

Weight Gain: Sometimes a person gains weight unexpectantly. Since too much weight is bad for your health, look for a reason. Because usually short-term memory is impaired (what one remembers about what happened recently), some people cannot remember they have eaten a meal. One lady living in a nursing facility would insist she did not get breakfast and ask for a tray just 15 minutes after finishing her tray. If she asked someone who did not know she did this, she would get another tray. She did the same thing for lunch and dinner. It wasn't until we noticed how much weight she was gaining that we realized what was happening.

Potential Delirium Indicators: An acute infection, urinary tract infection, any condition which causes a person to suddenly become confused and which gets better after treatment or removal of the cause. Think of conditions as delirium if they there is a potential for getting better. If delirium is as a result of cardiac medication and the person will die without it, then deal with it as dementia because dealing with it as if it is delirium is not useful. See delirium sheet.

What have we tried? Look to see what methods worked before in managing this behavior. Write down antipsychotic, neuroleptic or antidepressant medications. We need to know how much is given, how often it is given as well as how long this person has been using this medication. It is important to count the number of behaviors also. One wants to know whether medication added makes the behavior better or worse. One lady, a nursing home resident had been combative and throwing pottery 12-14 times a month. The antipsychotic medication was increased, and then she started doing this behavior 12-14 times every two weeks. This is always harder to assess if the person is on more than one of these kind of medications because one cannot know which medication is making her worse. Also, one does not know how much of what is occurring is a side effect of medication or as a result of the biochemical changes brought about by many different medications.

ACTION Plan: After looking at all the factors, we decide what we believe will work best for right now. If we think delirium is a factor and there is a cause which can be removed, it may be a temporary action plan until we see the real dementia by curing the delirium. A person can have delirium and dementia at the same time. When he or she does, you are not dealing with the core behavior but still need something to do until delirium can be treated.

EXAMPLE OF A COMPLETED FORM

FACTORS TO CHECK FOR PRIOR TO BEHAVIOR MANAGEMENT

Name: John Woods   Room 207-A   Prior living: nursing facility

Pertinent Social History: Widowed. 1 son, retired from Ford Motor Company. Admitted to the nursing facility 9-23   Age: 87

Diagnoses: Post open reduction internal fixation left hip fracture; hypothyroidism, Hyperglycemia; History -TB, emphysema, & pneumonia

___**Impaired Speech**   ✓ **Difficulty Understanding** ___**HOH** ___**Vision Problem**
Observed Behavior: Respiratory distress as a result of anxiety over fear he will not receive his pain medication complicated by diminished lung capacity. Long term use of Valium to relieve respiratory symptoms.

How long has the behavior been occurring? Since return from the hospital

Does behavior occur No BEFORE eating No AFTER eating No Shift Change

Medications which may affect behavior? Digoxin, Thyroid

Abnormal Lab: 9/10 urinalysis= +2 bacteria, 3+blood [urinary tract infection]; 9/15 BUN 33[indicator of increased fluid need] CO2 elevated 8=9/18 albumin low 2.8 [indicating a nutritional potential for skin problems.

Cardiovascular: Ischemic heart disease; history of atrial fibrillation; pacemaker status; History of bradycardia; mitral valve regurgitation; moderately severe aortic stenosis.

Respiratory: Pulmonary hypertension, possible acute process; possible neoplasm, patchy infiltrates; superimposed acute process; late effect TB cannot be ruled out; Chronic Obstructive Pulmonary Disease. Reported history of Valium used to maintain respiratory function.

Urinary Tract Problems: Urinary tract infection being treated, awaiting follow up urinalysis.

Pain Evidence: 9/24 respiratory distress - not wanting to eat; wedge compression deformities of several thoracic vertebrae - so needs to be kept off back & position changed to prevent pain; osteopenia; recent surgery hip fracture; scoliosis spine; pelvis osteopenic.

Hydration: Elevated BUN; at risk skin breakdown, urinary tract infection, elevated sodium, diminished bowel sounds all 4 quadrants at time of admission.

Weight Loss/Gain: admission weight 95.4 - very low

Potential Delirium Indicators: urinary tract infection, thyroid, Digoxin use, respiratory difficulties, potential malnutrition, potential dehydration

What have we tried? Increasing Valium which resulted in decline in ability to eat and increase in lethargy. Valium reduced to pre-hospital levels resulting in being better able to communicate with him.

ACTION Plan: Ask DR to evaluate- urinary tract infection status, increasing hydration, pain prevention. Nurse to bring his pain medication right before due time. Keep a list of time pills given at bedside for him to "see" pills are given on time - reassure him.

NAME: _____ Room: _____ DATE: _____
BEHAVIOR RECOMMENDATIONS   FROM: _____
OBSERVED BEHAVIOR: _____
_____
_____
_____
_____

HOW LONG HAS BEHAVIOR BEEN OCCURRING? _____
_____

PROBLEMS NOTED WITH:
_____ABNORMAL LAB   _____
_____CARDIAC_____
_____
_____
_____RESPIRATORY _____
_____
_____
_____HYDRATION _____
_____WEIGHT LOSS _____
_____ROOMMATE _____
_____ARTHRITIS _____
_____VISION _____
_____HEARING _____
_____AFTER EATING _____
_____BEFORE EATING _____
_____OTHER _____
WE TRIED: _____
ASSOCIATED DIAGNOSES: _____   _____
REQUEST PERMISSION TO:
_____
_____
_____
_____

ATTENDING PHYSICIAN REPLY: ____ACCEPTABLE ___NOT
COMMENTS:

DATE: _____ DR SIGNATURE:_____

Deborah A. Bastedo

EXAMPLE

NAME ___John Woods___ Room: __207-A__ DATE __10-1-98__

BEHAVIOR RECOMMENDATIONS   FROM: ___charge nurse___

OBSERVED BEHAVIOR: Anxiety shown by yelling in a loud and angry voice and continuing to do so until he receives his pain medication Respiratory distress 4 times a day as a result of anxiety over fear he will not receive his pain medication complicated by diminished lung capacity

HOW LONG HAS BEHAVIOR BEEN OCCURRING? Since admission____

PROBLEMS NOTED WITH:

_X_ ABNORMAL LAB 9/10 UA 2+bacteria; 9/15 BUN 33; 9/18 albumin low 2.8
_X_ CARDIAC Ischemic heart disease; hx atrial fib; pacemaker; mitral valve regurg moderately severe aortic stenosis. Hx of bradycardia.
_X_ RESPIRATORY Pulmonary hypertension; poss. acute process, poss. neoplasm patchy infiltrates; superimposed acute process; TB cannot be ruled out; COPD
_X_ HYDRATION diminished bowel sounds X4 on admission; UTI: at risk skin break down
_X_ WEIGHT LOSS low weight on admit -95.4
___ ROOMMATE _____
_X_ ARTHRITIS 9/24 resp distress - not wanting to eat; compression deformities T vertebrae -osteopenia -recent surgery hip fracture; scoliosis
___ VISION _____
___ HEARING _____
___ AFTER EATING _____
___ BEFORE EATING _____
_X_ OTHER On Valium for respiratory distress_____
WE TRIED: Valium for distress and **reactive** pain medication._____
ASSOCIATED DIAGNOSES: pulmonary hypertension, patchy infiltrates late effect of TB cannot be ruled out

REQUEST PERMISSION TO:

1. 1. Use **preventive** pain management strategy to lessen anxiety and prevent distress.
2. To increase hydration by giving 8 oz water at each time medication given
3. To improve nutritional status by giving high protein supplement 3 times a day and a multivitamin daily to enhance nutritional status

ATTENDING PHYSICIAN REPLY: _____ACCEPTABLE _____NOT

COMMENTS:

58

BEHAVIOR TRACKING:

The purpose of behavior tracking is to identify and write down what happened directly before inappropriate behavior occurred. Remember a person with dementia no longer has good judgment. He/she no longer understands it is not okay to do things such as take off all his/her clothes in front of others. This person no longer understands it is wrong to hit someone. The part of the brain which makes judgments and understands the rules for interacting with others is impaired by dementia. It is not defiance, it is dementia.

Caregivers can keep a list or use a blank piece of paper. A behavior tracking record form is presented later in this chapter which provides reminders of some things to note. This is especially important if a dementia victim's behavior changes suddenly. Tracking behavior can be one way of looking for patterns which will make caregiving an easier task.

What is the behavior tracking record? The behavior tracking record is a list of what we have learned by working with this demented person. The purpose of tracking the person's behavior is to learn from what this person does in order to prevent behavior which is not appropriate in the future. If we notice that moving her dresser upsets her, then we can prevent her being upset by not moving her dresser.

Just as in poker, what good players look for are "tells," meaning mannerisms or behavior which tells them when the other person is bluffing. Tracking inappropriate behavior can also help us learn this person's "tells." Does he or she wiggle or say "oh oh" right before soiling himself. Sometimes caregivers make a list of the times a person eliminates in order to encourage them to sit on the toilet before the time this person usually has an accident. In this way the caregiver may be able to prevent accidents.

Often if we ask a demented person if he is in pain, he will say "no." Then he will proceed to groan and hold his belly or chest. Just as demented people no longer remember what to do, they also do not remember what words mean, such as "pain." My father complained of chest pain when in the emergency room of the hospital. I summoned the doctor who asked him if he was in pain. He said, "no." By the time I could get the doctor to believe he was in pain, he had had a heart attack. Pain is a very important aspect of care to track. Since strong medications are not good for people unless needed, we can identify what this person does which tells you he/she is in pain. Hopefully if we watch what a person does and identify the cause of the pain, then we will be able to prevent it or at least treat it when it needs treating. For example, let's say that Martha Jones is grimacing, meaning she is in pain. Because we know that for her this is low-level pain, we can give her a less strong pain medication such as Tylenol or Motrin. But let's say she is in a fetal position. Now for her we have noted that this means she is in a lot of pain. For this behavior we might give a stronger medication for pain; or if we know this is for arthritis pain, we could use an anti-inflammatory drug if doctor has prescribed one. Since dementia victims may no longer be able to tell us they hurt, we have to watch for their "tells."

BEHAVIOR TRACKING RECORD

Name:_____

Likes to be called:_____

Is vision impaired?_____ **Hearing**_____

What type of voice works best?

Friendly? _____ **Soft spoken?**_____ **FIRM?**_____

Are there any words which make him/her feel better?_____

_____

Names of family/friends?_____

What makes him/her perk up? Singing? ___ **Silence?**____ **TV off?** ____ **Other** _____

Does she like Touch_____ **Massage**_____ **Music**_____, **what kind?**_____

_____

What upsets him/her?_____

_____

What does this person do which means: Pain scale 1-10 (10 worst)

In pain?_____

COLD? _____ **HUNGRY?**_____

WET? _____ **OVER STIMULATED?** _____

AFRAID?_____

OTHER? _____

_____

COMMENTS:_____

_____

_____

_____

DATE: _____**SIGNATURE:** _____

BEHAVIOR TRACKING RECORD   (example)

Name: __Martha Jones___   Likes to be called: __"grandma"___

Is her vision impaired?_ Yes but okay with glasses Hearing? Slightly hard of hearing

What type of voice works best? friendly _√_   soft spoken ____   firm___   other:_____Are there any words which make him/her feel better? _"It's okay not to remember things – we all forget sometimes."___

_____

Names of family/friends: _Cindy (granddaughter) Hazel (next door neighbor)_

What makes him/her perk up? singing? √   silence?_√_ TV off?_ Noisy situations   upset   her   – she's a people person but only in small groups or 1 to 1._____

Does she like: Touch?__Massage?____ Music?____What kind? Church music_____

What upsets him/her?_   Loud confusing situations, large groups of people slow down   her   ability   to function and she cannot do everything she can otherwise do_____

WHAT DOES THIS PERSON DO WHICH MEANS: Pain scale 1-10 (10 worst)

In pain?_____1-3 grimaces; 4-6 holding chest or abdomen; 7-8 fights with caregivers; 9-10 curls up in fetal position_____ **HUNGRY?**sits at table even if not meal time_____

COLD?_____Says, "it hurts, it hurts" (becomes quiet when blanket or sweater put on_____

WET? Wiggles and says "Oh Oh Oh" **OVER STIMULATED:** more confused_____

AFRAID? Goes to bed, withdraws_____

OTHER?_ When her personal things are moved (esp. the dresser) she gets extremely upset – it is very important that no one moves the things in her room._____

COMMENTS:_   1/12/02 had a urinary tract infection became more confused and acted out by hitting others, better after antibiotics. 2/10/02 had bronchitis became more   confused   but   better   after antibiotics; 2/23/02 dresser moved for cleaning became very upset, yelling; When asked if she is in pain – she always says, "no"- need to watch her   actions to decide if she is in pain.

The next page is an outline of factors to remember to check for prior to even considering the use of an antipsychotic drug. It was developed from Michigan surveyor comments. It should be noted that in contrast to antipsychotic medication, antidepressant medication can be effective in making the person more capable with fewer side effects. In fact, in terms of survey for long term care facilities, use of antidepressants is considered a positive indicator (credit for good care.)

BASED ON NURSING FACILITY FEDERAL CRITERIA

WHEN IS IT OKAY TO ASK FOR AN ORDER FOR ANTIPSYCHOTIC MEDICATIONS?

!!!ONLY AS A LAST RESORT!!!

Behavior problems are especially common with **antipsychotic medications.**
The medical record must contain documented evidence the nursing facility staff checked EVERYTHING ELSE FIRST!

Documentation should include but not be limited to:

What happened that might trigger the behavior?

        NEW ROOMMATE?
        NEW TO NURSING HOME?
        DID THE PERSON ARGUE WITH A FAMILY MEMBER?
        DID THE PERSON JUST HAVE A DEATH IN THE FAMILY?
Look for **abnormal lab work** and tests.

        Does urinalysis indicate bacteria? Positive nitrite? Urinary tract infection?
        Does complete blood count indicate low hemoglobin, anemia?
        Does chest x-ray show pneumonia or degenerative bone disease?
Look for **respiratory symptoms.**

        Write down lung sounds. Were they the same as when last assessed?
        How do the lungs sound?

Is this person on **a new medication?**
        Side effects?   Narcotic?   Strong?
Is this person on MULTIPLE medications? COULD THEY BE INTERACTING?
IS THIS PERSON **IN PAIN**? Does the behavior happen during dressing, grooming or bathing? When assisting him from chair or out of bed? Is there a gentler way to help him which does not involve moving or pulling on joints too much? Can DR recommend pain management?
Is there evidence of an **INFECTION?** ANYWHERE in the person's body? Can be teeth or toes or skin or nose or bladder, etc.
Is there evidence of **dehydration?** sunken eyes, pale, red lips, crease in tongue, concentrated urine, big weight loss over short time - like 8 pounds in a week, BUN of 23 or above means more fluid needed unless caused by a diagnosed condition.
Is there evidence of **cardiac problems?** Abnormal EKG? Is it being treated?
BEHAVIOR MANAGEMENT. LOOK for what causes the behavior (what triggers it). In what way can you tell the person is going to do the behavior? Does he start by grunting, then end up by hitting? How often, where and when does behavior occur? Then what works in controlling it and what does NOT work. FOCUS ON THE PERSON'S STRENGTHS AND WHAT HE OR SHE **CAN** DO AND **NEVER** STOP TRYING.

IN ORDER FOR A PERSON TO BE A CANDIDATE FOR ANTIPSYCHOTIC MEDICATION, THERE MUST BE DOCUMENTED EVIDENCE OF LONG TERM PSYCHIATRIC HISTORY AND/OR SEVERE MENTAL ILLNESS DIAGNOSIS.

Chapter 16

DEMENTIA LANGUAGE TRANSLATOR

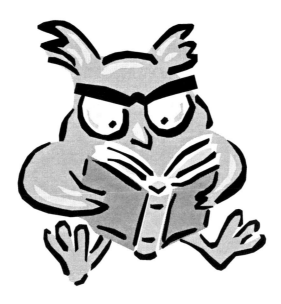

When we speak with a person with dementia, we need to remember he or she is doing his or her best to communicate.

What is this person trying to tell us with his/her behavior and actions?

ATTACHMENT

In <u>Development Through Life A Psychosocial Approach</u> (p. 203), the author defines infant attachment as "An attachment is... an internal representation of the characteristics of a specific relationship... provides the infant (demented person) with a set of rules with which to organize information and to interpret experiences(.)" This is exactly what I see when observing confused people. Often you will see a confused person follow the person who is their security person around as though they are glued to that person.

This can result in a large range of behavior which is difficult. - I found that using solutions which would work on a 2-year-old also worked on Dad.

Such as: Hitting and Screaming behavior

For the lady who would go berserk when a familiar dresser was moved to clean under it, my solution was either not to clean under it or to move it when she was out of the room and put it back before she returned.

"My wife is dead and I don't know what to do."

He knew his wife wasn't with him and he could not remember where she was. Anxious behavior resulted. Since he could not see her, he was afraid. We got him a notebook and his wife wrote in it every time she visited. She would also write when she was coming back. So when he couldn't remember, caregivers could look it up for him.

"Can't you see the spacemen in the orange suit?"

I need you to confirm my world. If you do not see the spacemen, then the only thing I feel certain of is not correct and this is too upsetting for me right now. I need something I can hang onto, even if it is not true.

Possible answer: "Okay" or "So, there are spacemen outside your window. What are they doing?"

GENERAL SITUATIONS

"NO" This word is really tricky because it has so many different meanings.

If Dad continued the task - it meant "okay."

If Dad was showing me facial and body language symbols for refusal, probably "no" means, "I do not understand and this is scary to me."

If regarding a bath, it ALWAYS meant NO.

"The President came to see me today!" This means, "I heard his voice on TV." A psychiatrist wrote this person was hallucinating. However, this occurred directly before a presidential election and this person was almost blind. The president's voice on TV sounded every bit as real as the people in the hallway to him. This is not hallucinating, it is poor vision.

HITTING - SOME CAUSES

Could be a deaf person, grabbed from behind.
Grabbing a person by an arthritic shoulder to help him or her. Grabbing a person by the shoulder who has had trauma to that shoulder - especially if he or she has a torn rotator cuff.
Startling a person who fears being assaulted.
Pain - Is the person showing pain symptoms (see chapter on pain)
Trying to force a confused person to do something.
Fear that being touched will result in pain.

ARGUING with a demented person will OFTEN result in aggressive action.

LOST

"I gotta pee and it won't come out."
I have to urinate and I cannot remember where the bathroom is, OR
I am wet, OR I no longer know what the toilet "looks" like. Making the toilet seat a contrasting color can help people "see" the toilet. Often bathrooms are all white or light colors. The changes mentally and visually which occur make "seeing" the toilet difficult.
Sometimes a person will be searching for something. He/she does not know what they are searching for but think that if they find it, they will know what it is.
Nothing looks familiar to them.

PAIN BEHAVIOR

crying and tearfulness hitting people
removing clothing - especially pants or skirts
grimacing, frowning - refusing to cooperate with daily care help
"It hurts, it hurts!" I believe that if you touch me it is going to hurt.

"A caregiver slapped me." My cheek hurts and I do not know why. (Federal studies show that if a demented person says it hurts—it probably does hurt somewhere.)

SEX

"There are a lot of bad people here. I saw them having sex in the hallway all night. Not being able to see very well. This lady had macular degeneration (deterioration of ability to see) and was almost blind. When she was in bed at night, shadows in the hallway "looked like" sex to her cause she could not make them out.

"Two women raped me, one held me down, and the other raped me."
This woman had soiled herself and her caregivers were giving her a bed bath.

SHOWERS

"You are hurting me with all these pins."
The water feels like pins to me. Research indicates the changes in the brain as a result of dementia also affect the senses. So the sense of taste and smell and touch as well as sight and hearing all may be affected. The water really does feel like pins and needles. Dad did this; we gave him tub baths or bed baths.
Screaming in shower -"Why are you are picking me with needles?"
Early dementia language: Means sense of touch impaired - the water in the shower really does feel like needles to the demented person. So give him a bath instead.
Screaming in shower -"Why are you are poking me with toothpicks?"
Later dementia language: Means sense of touch impaired. The water in the shower really does feel like toothpicks to the demented person. Give him a bath instead.

TASTE CHANGES

"Someone is poisoning my food!" "They only feed me nuts and bolts." Food doesn't taste the same anymore. I do not like to eat and when I do eat, it tastes awful.

TOILET PROBLEMS

Smearing bowel movement all over. Could be hemorrhoids, constipation, or the desire to be touched. Could also be a partial memory related to a time when he or she did art work and not having intact judgment to know what her art medium is or that the world sees this as gross.

WANDERING

"My wife is coming to get me soon."
"I cannot find my home."

I want to go home. This place does not seem familiar like home to me (even if it is my home): I need some familiar things, which I recognize and familiar faces around me. This person may not feel like where he is home <u>as he remembers home to be</u>. Perhaps family pictures or a picture of him or a familiar chair or a box full of pictures and familiar objects (a memory box) might help.

See if you can tell what "caused" this person to wander. There was a lady would try to leave her nursing facility every day at 3:30 p.m. It turns out she used to work day shift at General Motors. At 3:30 p.m. when she saw day shift nursing facility staff put on their coats, she thought it was time to go home.

When I speak with demented people, they will indicate they need to be somewhere but do not know where. I saw my role as one of helping them find a destination. It may seem impossible to get someone to stop wandering. Dad would be responding to pain sometimes. If I gave him a pain reliever, he might sit down and relax.

DEMENTIA

SELF

TEST*

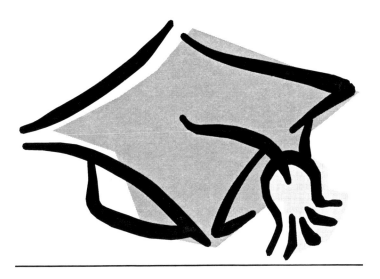

*An answer key follows but please remember the dialect for the language of dementia is *different* FOR EACH PERSON, which means the same phrase or action may mean different things for different people.

Dementia Questionnaire - What does it feel like to have dementia?

1. What is dementia?

2. What is delirium?

3. How can you tell the difference?

4. Can a person have both dementia and delirium at the same time?

5. Once a person has Alzheimer's Disease, they no longer have feelings like everyone.
       True   or   False

6. Forgetfulness is a normal part of aging. True or False

7. Match the reaction with the possible causes for what a dementia person feels.

screams in shower, dementia	hemorrhoids
screams in shower, dementia	constipated
macular degeneration [vision impairment]	people having sex in the hallway
changes in taste sensations	desire to be touched
floaters in the visual field	There are bugs all over the wall
misperception due to elevated blood sugar	Can't you see the orange space men?
smearing BM all over	needles, hitting my skin
smearing BM all over	deaf-grabbed from behind
smearing BM all over	toothpicks hitting my skin
hitting caregivers	Someone is poisoning my food.
hitting caregivers	grabbed by shoulder [torn rotator cuff]
hitting caregivers	startled, hearing impaired, approached from behind

8. Match the dementia statements with a possible NON demented translation:

"It hurts, it hurts"	My privates were cleaned and I DID NOT understand.
"A caregiver slapped me"	My sense of taste is impaired.
"It hurts, it hurts"	If you touch me, it will hurt.
"Two women raped me, one held me down, and the other..."	I am cold.
"It hurts, it hurts"	My cheek hurt and I could not remember why.
"They only feed me nuts and bolts"	I heard the president on TV
"The president came to see me today"	I am in pain

9. When a person with dementia cries, caregivers do not ALWAYS look for pain.

   True or False.   Is there pain?

10. In order to best help this person, we need to keep our approach simple, kind, loving, and reassuring. Look for solutions thinking of a 2-year old in a 6-foot body, but with the respect one would show a venerated elder. True or False

Dementia Questionnaire - What does it feel like to have dementia?

ANSWER KEY

1. What is dementia? **A slowly worsening brain disease noticed by changes in behavior and personality changes and by a decline in ability to think. Not reversible**

2. What is delirium? **A SUDDEN mental status change which is usually reversible.**

3. How can you tell the difference? **If you can cure the sudden change by treating a health problem then it is delirium.**

4. Can a person have both dementia and delirium at the same time? **YES**

5. Once a person has Alzheimer's Disease, they no longer have feelings like everyone.
   False

6. Forgetfulness is a normal part of aging. True or False
   False

7. <u>Match the reaction with the possible causes for what a dementia person feels.</u>

screams in shower, dementia———————	toothpicks hitting my skin
screams in shower, dementia———————	needles, hitting my skin
macular degeneration [vision impairment]——	people having sex in the hallway
changes in taste sensations———————	Someone is poisoning my food.
floaters in the visual field———————	There are bugs all over the wall
misperception due to elevated blood sugar——	Can't you see the orange space men?
smearing BM all over———————	hemorrhoids
smearing BM all over———————	constipated
smearing BM all over———————	desire to be touched
hitting caregivers———————	deaf-grabbed from behind
hitting caregivers————————	grabbed by shoulder [torn rotator cuff]
hitting caregivers———————	startled, hearing impaired, approached from behind

8. <u>Match the dementia statements with a possible NON demented translation:</u>

"A caregiver slapped me"———————	My cheek hurt and I could not remember why.
"It hurts, it hurts"———————	I am in pain
"Two women raped me, one held me down, and the other..."	My privates were cleaned and I DID NOT understand.
"It hurts, it hurts"———————	I am cold.
"They only feed me nuts and bolts"———————	My sense of taste is impaired.
"The president came to see me today."———	I heard the president on TV

9. When a person with dementia cries, caregivers do not ALWAYS look for pain.
   True   Is there pain? **YES, PROBABLY THERE IS**

10. In order to best help this person, we need to keep our approach simple, kind, loving, and reassuring. Look for solutions thinking of a 2-year old in a 6-foot body, but with the respect one would show a venerated elder. **True**

Chapter 17

BEHAVIOR MANAGEMENT

PLANS FOR CARE*

*Please note this section is based on nursing facility care but contains many good ideas for use in any living environment. Abbreviations used:

ACT - Activities
SW - Social service staff
RD - Registered Dietitian
DIET - dietary

DR - Physician
CNA - Caregiver
NSG - Nurse
esp. - especially

These care plans are based on actual residents in a nursing home setting. The names as well as any facts which would be identifying have been changed to preserve the privacy of the person about whom they were written. They are intended as "ideas." Each demented person is different and will react as an individual.

The most important part of determining a care plan is focusing on "what works." No matter how pretty something "sounds," abandon it for what works and you will do so much better in managing difficult behavior.

"Mary Martin" is the care plan written from a surveyor citation and was viewed and "approved" for compliance by a Michigan surveyor.

Deborah A. Bastedo

Index of Behavior REASONS By Fictitious Person's Name

ARGUING
Joseph Marsac
Mary Martin

CHOICES - DESIRE TO MAKE CHOICES
Ray Coleman
Joseph Marsac
Mary Martin

COMMUNICATION IMPAIRMENT
Alexis Bastedo
Catherine Berdan
Laurence Fuller
Marilyn Hayden

FEAR/ANXIETY
Catherine Berdan
Laurence Fuller
Joseph Marsac

FIGHTING WITH FAMILY
Frances Smith

HARD OF HEARING
Ray Coleman
Frances Smith

LOSS OF INDEPENDENCE
Laurence Fuller
Frances Smith

LOST ROLES
Alexis Bastedo
Ray Coleman
Frances Smith
Beth Stickney

NO FAMILY
Ethel Woods

SAD/DEPRESSED
Geri Bentfield
Karen Patillo
Frances Smith
Beth Stickney

CHRONIC PAIN
Alexis Bastedco
Geri Bentfield
Catherine Berdan
Marilyn Hayden
Joseph Marsac
Karen Patillo
Mabel Renshaw
Frances Smith
Beth Stickney
Ethel Woods

Too much Medication - Dizzy
Beth Stickney

SOCIALLY INAPPROPRIATE
Ray Coleman
Laurence Fuller
Ethel Woods

SHOWER SCARY
Mabel Renshaw

PHYSICALLY AGGRESSIVE
Laurence Fuller

VERBALLY ABUSIVE
Ray Coleman
Karen Patillo
Ethel Woods

MISSES TOILET
Beth Stickney

POOR VISION
Catherine Berdan
Ray Coleman
Ethel Woods

WANDERING
Catherine Berdan
Marilyn Hayden
Karen Patillo

Deborah A. Bastedo

Editor:

Behavior Management Plan

Behavior Trigger [cause of behavior]	Behavior	What works [Approaches]	Goals
Physical & Emotional Pain Desire to make choices over her care—life. Feeling of hopelessness—resulting in resistance to EVERYTHING as her way of making choices. 46 year old in nursing home with lack of activity which would be meaningful for her age. Rejection of people as she believes she has been rejected. SADNESS over lost role in community as daughter, wife, desirable female.	Physically abusive 1-3 days in 7. Kicking primarily 7 am to 3 pm. Hitting 7 am to 11 pm. Biting primarily 7 am to 3 pm—7/98. Daily ANGER Easily annoyed. Verbally abusive 1-3 days in 7. Refuses to sit in hallway.	**DR** and **NSG** to evaluate complicating issues to resolve if possible. TRY routine pain RX esp. 20 min before moving her before AM care before PM care before Therapy. ALL to ask her permission before doing ANYTHING to her. Allow her to choose to do tasks later. Offer her at least 2 options. **ACT** to identify more meaningful **activities** + Look for peer group which might visit or other volunteer visitors. Try **cosmetics** to see if this makes her feel more "normal." Dress her in **street clothing** so she looks more "normal?"	Resolve complicating issues Anticipate and prevent pain. Verbal abuse will reduce to 2 times a week or less. Kicking & hitting will reduce to 3 times a week or less. Biting will cease and will not reoccur. Provide pain relief & diversions to avoid anger. Each shift will have some activity other than radio for her diversion. She will make choices at least 3 times a day.

NAME: **Alexis Bastedo**   Room number: **214B**   Case number: Date: Signature

Person's Strengths: She can communicate, she wishes to make choices, family supportive

Behavior Management Plan

Behavior Trigger [cause of behavior]	Behavior	What works [Approaches]	Goals
.**Cannot think of words to say.** **Complications** **Clouding judgement** **PAIN subflexed shoulder Ext. contraction Potential urinary tract infect** **Low potassium** **Chronic constipation** **Brain misfires** due to previous brain surgery— **Thalmic bleed** **On Potent medications** with possible side effects	Resists care 4-6 days in 7. Daily exposes buttocks lying in almost fetal position with her head toward her radio.	SW to assist in finding word board or picture board so that when she cannot find the correct words so she has choices other than swearing. **ALL** caregivers leave room when negative behavior—do not give a response-offer simple choices such as between two gowns or allow her to choose to 'do it later' **Praise cooperation** **DIET** provide nutritional support—Adjust diet to avoid constipation without medication if possible Minimize pain—maintain muscle strength Get her to 'want' to behave by having staff pay more attention for good behaviors **rather** than bad.	Physical abuse will reduce to 2 times a week or less. Better communication **Staff will** pay more attention to her during times when behavior is acceptable. She will no longer expose her buttocks. **Radio** will not be her only interest.

NAME: **Alexis Bastedo**   Room number: **214B**   Case number: Date: Signature

Person's Strengths: She can communicate, she wishes to make choices, family supportive

Behavior Management Plan

Behavior Trigger [cause of behavior]	Behavior	What works [Approaches]	Goals
Hard of hearing misses part of the message	Frequently crying. Withdrawal from activity and people.	**ALL** speak clearly and VERY LOUD but calm, use 4 word sentences. REPEAT & REPEAT what you say. Offer 1 or 2 choices. **ACT** provide activities which do not depend on good hearing.	Resident will understand part of message q shift daily Res. will have busy schedule during waking hours
Lack of activities meaningful to her.		**SW** get hearing evaluated **ALL** touch her before moving her or providing care. **SW** to help her make friends with other women who have lost husbands.	Prevent pain and fear during care encounters
Major Depression Husband's death. 9/9 denies depression	Grief relative to death of husband. Frequent crying. Poor appetite. Weight loss.	**ACT** to visit & encourage. **DIET** to review nutritional status and recommend. **Family** to visit 3 times a week and provide emotional support.	She will have one or more peers with whom to vent. She will consume 75% or more of her diet.

NAME: **Geri Bentfield**   Room number: **205-3**   Case number: Date: Signature

Person's Strengths: Desire to communicate with others; supportive family; desire to make choices.

Deborah A. Bastedo

Behavior Management Plan

Behavior Trigger [cause of behavior]	Behavior	What works [Approaches]	Goals Complicating
Admitted on Stelazine unable to obtain reason from Hospital? **No long term history of mental illness?** 6/23 Pneumonia 7/31 Urinary Tract Infection (UTI) 9/23 Stelazine reduced **Complications:** PAIN severe Degenerative Joint Disease (DJD); Compression Fracture L1 vertebrae Status post surgery—nephrectomy.	Agitated, angry outbursts daily. Pain relative to recent surgery and symptomatic DJD, UTI, back pain during first 30-45 days of stay.	**DR** to eval to see if symptoms as a result of complicating problems such as pneumonia. **DR** will identify & treat complicating problems **DR** and **Psych DR** will evaluate and reduce Stelazine if possible. **DR** to assess for medication within the guidelines of HCFA **Pastoral Minister visits** **DR & NSG** to assess for pain & treat proactively. **Staff to** anticipate her needs. USE arthritis approach—gentle encourage her not to remain in position against spine for longer than 2 hours **Family** to bring in arthritis-friendly clothing with Velcro closures.	problems will be eliminated. **Reduce** angry outbursts to 3 times a week or less. **Reduce** and/or discontinue Stelazine. **Anticipate & Prevent** pain, allowing maximum quality of life. **Promote** her assisting in her daily care.

NAME: **Geri Bentfield**   Room number: **205-3**   Case number: Date: Signature
Person's Strengths: Desire to communicate with others; supportive family; desire to make choices.

Behavior Management Plan

Behavior Trigger [cause of behavior]	Behavior	What works [Approaches]	Goals
Cerebral atrophy complicated by: Vision impairment which causes her to misperceive her environment [wears glasses]. **Pain limits range of motion**	Talks to furniture. Can be aggressive. Resists getting dressed, groomed, bathed daily.	**ALL** make sure she has her glasses—Touch her before you begin care Increase lighting in her room but avoid glare. **DR-NSG** to assess cause of pain & how she shows pain & prevent pain—esp. morning & bedtime care & before therapy & ADL esp. bathing **Caregivers** to use arthritis friendly techniques by not pulling or lifting her joints	**She** will gain calm from gentle touch. **She** will not be startled **She** will be able to find a way to accommodate her misperceptions of the world using touch or written words. **Family** will bring in arthritis friendly clothes **She** will allow daily care. **Staff** will use gently touch & not extend extremities into painful reach. **Staff** will encourage her to help with daily care in order to minimize pain.

NAME: **Catherine Berdan**   Room number: **236-1**   Case number: Date: Signature

Person's Strengths: She can walk, desire to keep self busy, gets exercise; walks daily

Behavior Management Plan

Behavior Trigger [cause of behavior]	Behavior	What works [Approaches]	Goals
Cerebral atrophy Unable to comprehend what is said to her. Noisy confused areas reduce her ability to understand. FEAR of unknown complicated by Alzheimer-type dementia.	She becomes aggressive and yells daily. **Tearfulness daily.**	**DR** eval hearing & assess possible delirium causes to see if treatment is needed. REPEAT & REPEAT what you are saying. Try writing words down to see if she understands in this way. Approach her from the front. **ALL** need to keep a consistent routine— need to keep her out of noisy places. Use short clear 4 word phrases. Place her picture + her name in big letters on the door to her room. **FAMILY** to bring in memory box; make tape of family voices, bring in notebook to use as a visit log-family pictures.	**DR** will treat potential delirium causes. **She** will understand part of message being communicated. **Reduce** aggressive episodes to 3 times a week or less. **Reduce** tearfulness to 3 times a week or less. **She** will have the security of a consistent routine. Help her find her room. Provide homelike room.

NAME: **Catherine Berdan**   Room number: **236-1**   Case number: Date: Signature
Person's Strengths: She can walk, desire to keep self busy, gets exercise; walks daily

Behavior Management Plan

Behavior Trigger [cause of behavior]	Behavior	What works [Approaches]	Goals
Not enough for her to do.

Hx-factory worker VFW member. | Wanders into other people's rooms daily.

8/5—She shut off the light in another person's room & he hit, scratched & swore at her. | **ACT** need her to have objects to manipulate + quiet room where she can wander and "touch" things.

ACT try confusion board with lights and/or light switch. | **Reduce** wandering to 3 times a week or less.

She will have a safe space to walk around where she will not bother anyone else.

She will have something familiar to manipulate. |

NAME: **Catherine Berdan**   Room number: **236-1**   Case number: Date: Signature

Person's Strengths: She can walk, desire to keep self busy, gets exercise; walks daily

Behavior Management Plan

Behavior Trigger	Behavior	What works	Goals
[cause of behavior]	Crying daily.	[Approaches]	**Reduce** crying to every other day or eliminate it.
Major DEPRESSION	"I want to be dead." per 6/26 psych. evaluation.	Psych. DR to continue.	
		ACT to provide alternatives to medication for anxiety relief.	**She** will consume 75% or more of her food.
Rectal mass—pathology negative for cancer.	Also makes anxious statements; negative statements; repetitive statements.	**Staff** to pay more attention to her when she is not anxious.	To **encourage** venting rather than anxious statements.
Colostomy status stool trapped between colostomy & rectum complicated by HYPODYNAMIC ILEUS		**Family** to visit & make a tape with family voices to make her room more like home & bring in familiar objects—pictures of family	Her room will feel more, "like home."
Lost role grade school teacher.	Wants to stay in bed all the time.	**ACT** to pair her up with a friend who used to be a schoolteacher.	
Pattern of weight loss.		**Pastoral Minister** visits.	
		SW to provide visitation and to reassure & find her a friend who has a colostomy.	**PM** to assist her in accepting her health status and coming to terms with her spiritual beliefs.
		DIET to provide supplement, additional fluids, and health shakes with meals as well as additional fiber.	**DIET** to monitor nutritional status and help prevent dehydration and pressure ulcers. Praise calm responses.

NAME: **Mary Coleman**   Room number: **202-4**   Case number: Date: **9-30**   Signature

Person's Strengths: Desire to be free from pain; desire to make choices

Behavior Management Plan

Behavior Trigger	Behavior	What works	Goals
[cause of behavior] Almost Deaf on left. Vision impaired on left. 4/12 ischemic infart 6/22 abnormal EKG Cardiomegaly Chronic Obstructive Pulmonary Disease. 9/13 Urinary Tract Infection- per hospital. PAIN—osteoporosis spine—esp. Thoracic Tends to get pressure ulcers.	Crying daily. Says in pain then refuses pain medicine.	[Approaches] **DR** to evaluate potential for dehydration. **All** approach her from right. & USE GENTLE HAPPY VOICE. MAKE EYE CONTACT on each encounter. Be gentle in your approach. Do NOT tug or pull on arms & legs. Offer simple choices. Preventive pain management. Very important as has been cause of anxiety **NSG** to assess non verbal sign of pain due to her difficulty understanding & monitor lung sounds for changes & bowel sounds for changes. **ACT** to play relaxing cassette tapes & meditation tapes for her.	**Reduce** crying to every other day or eliminate it. **DR** to resolve acute process and resolvable conditions. She will choose time for pain medicine. **ALL STAFF** to encourage pain prevention & prevent pain by changes in positioning and calm, relaxing environment. **She** will be pressure sore free.

NAME: **Mary Coleman**   Room number: **202-4**   Case number: Date: **9-30**   Signature

Person's Strengths: Desire to be free from pain; desire to make choices

Behavior Management Plan

Behavior Trigger	Behavior	What works	Goals
[cause of behavior] Physical pain.	Tearful—emotional pain	[Approaches] **DR** to assess for cause & effective routine pain medicine to be given before AM & bedtime care & before restorative nursing or therapy	Provide effective pain management to prevent pain and the behavior problems that result from pain.
Thoracic vertebral (Spine) degeneration with resulting pain	VERBALLY ABUSIVE 1 to 3 days out of 5	**NSG** to identify dementia ways to indicate pain such as hits, kicks, swears - **tearful**	He will not be in the same position for longer than 2 hours.
Pain with movement esp. morning and evening care & when in same sitting position for longer than 2 hours	He grimaces and swears when he sits in the same position too long + when approached for care.	**CAREGIVER** Do not position him on Thoracic spine Use positioning pillows for comfort at bedtime Take him to toilet before he becomes wet.	He will vent his feelings without needing to yell or hit at staff daily.
Complications: NEEDS ASSISTANCE with bathing, dressing, grooming, going to toilet. Embarrassed when he wets himself.		Use gentle approach for all care—arthritis friendly—do not extend leg or arms beyond pain tolerance. **FAMILY** to get arthritis friendly clothing. (velcro rather than buttons.)	He will have friends who live there and visit him at least 3-5 times a week. Reduce verbal abuse to twice a week or less. Daily care will not hurt him.

NAME: **Raymond Coleman**   Room number: **351** Case number: Date: Signature
Person's Strengths: He can talk, He can help dress himself, family supportive, supportive visitors, desire to make choices

Behavior Management Plan

Behavior Trigger	Behavior	What works	Goals
[cause of behavior]	Hitting, swearing tearfulness.	[Approaches]	Help him find the positives in life role have him help in his own care.
Misperceives Environment & words with resulting fearful response because HARD OF HEARING and almost BLIND (MACULAR DEGENERATION)		DR to check for depression. Caregiver to use gentle approach + touch him before beginning care.	
	"I want to die."	SW to visit daily and encourage him to vent his feelings giving praise him for adaptive, positive words + to encourage community visitors.	Reduce socially inapprop activities to weekly or less often. ALL to offer him choices. Increase lighting in room. Use raised toilet seat for arthritis comfort.
9/3 POSS DEHYDRATION Loss identity—role of husband—father— community leader raised 5 own kids 2 wife's brothers ran farm member VFW volunteer DOES NOT KNOW WHERE HE FITS IN!	SOCIALLY INAPPROP 1 to 3 days out of 5		
	Territorial—hit & scratched man who entered his room.	ACT to help him find a friend with common interests. Family to bring in pictures and memory box with items he can feel.	Increase lighting to help limited sight + help prevent falls. Room will feel more like home.
	5/26 Increase in inappropriate behavior since 5/26 observed lying on floor.	ACT to encourage empowerment activities and keep him busy.	He will have activities to think about rather than his poor health daily.
	9/3 Decrease in understanding increase in hitting and swearing - does not make sense.	9/3 DR to assess. NSG to encourage fluids. RD to assess & recommend.	9/3 Dehydration will be healed as evidenced by a BUN of 22 or less.

NAME: **Raymond Coleman**　　Room number: **351**　　Case number:　　Date:　　Signature

Person's Strengths: He can talk, He can help dress himself, family supportive, supportive visitors, desire to make choices

Behavior Management Plan

Behavior Trigger [cause of behavior]	Behavior	What works [Approaches]	Goals
Anxiety over loss of possessions when confused people 'wander' into his room. "Territorial" Difficulty tolerating confused residents.

Anxiety over fear of dying (Younger sister died a year ago).

Poor impulse control due to major stroke. | Physically abusive 1 to 3 days out of 7. Verbally aggressive 1 to 3 days out of 7 when wanderers get in his way or come into his room.

Increase in physical aggressiveness.

Pushing people who get in his way. | 12-14 Psych evaluation suggests placing a Velcro piece of fabric from one door jam to the other. **DR** Trail use of Antidepressant unsuccessful discontinued. 7/30 Buspar begun— doing better.

Caregivers keep confused residents out of his path when wheeling down hall. | Keep other residents out of his room.

Reduce verbally and physically aggressive behavior to 1 to 2 times a week.

He will not push people who get in his way.

Keep confused people out of his way. |

NAME: **Laurence Fuller**   Room number: **201** Case number: Date: Signature

Person's Strengths: He can communicate, desire to make choices about his life, determination to be independent

Diagnoses: Chronic adjustment disorder with disturbance of conduct; poor impulse control; does not see inappropriate behavior as incorrect.

Behavior Management Plan

Behavior Trigger [cause of behavior]	Behavior	What works [Approaches]	Goals
Anxiety over fear of losing his independence complicated by poor balance and difficulty ambulating safely in a crowd of people. **Always lived alone** not accustomed to sharing living area ->Desire to eat in dining room in "his" chair **Slurred speech-** not understood by others. Too hard to communicate wish for more milk. Normal life long activity pattern self isolation.	Stabs people with fork if he/she try to get his food. Will take another residen't milk at lunch and dinner meals **DIET** will give him 2 milks on his trays	**Caregivers** to have him eat meals at a later time when fewer people in dining room -> placing one other resident at his table rather than 3 **ACT** to honor his choice to maintain his lifelong pattern of TV & Radio going at the same time as well as his refusal of all activities.	He will not stab people. Allow him to choose to eat in dining room three times a day in 'his' chair undisturbed. He will not need to take another person's milk.

NAME: **Laurence Fuller**   Room number: **201**   Case number: Date: Signature

Person's Strengths: He can communicate, desire to make choices about his life, determination to be independent

Diagnoses: Chronic adjustment disorder with disturbance of conduct; poor impulse control; does not see inappropriate behavior as incorrect.

Deborah A. Bastedo

Behavior Management Plan

Behavior Trigger [cause of behavior]	Behavior	What works [Approaches]	Goals
Disruption of ability to understand **verbal** communications—may miss part of message & misunderstands world around her resulting in **fear** and **anxious** responses. **Searching** for way to make words—world make sense.	May repeat words and try different ways to get whole message across. Fear response during verbal communication 3 or more times a day. Wanders 3 or more times daily—behavior not easily altered.	**ALL** make eye contact speak in short 4 word sentences—clear friendly voice. REPEAT & REPEAT **ALL** provide consistent routine daily **ACT** to provide dementia activity like busy hands or maybe let her set the tables in activities. Provide quiet area—try to reduce noise. Noise makes it harder for her to understand. Family to make visitor log so she can see when she had a visit. Help her find a friend she can help who can give her verbal reminders of what to do.	Provide non drug methods to reduce anxiety—gain comfort Reduce fear response to daily or less often. Reduce wandering to daily exercise **Maximize her understanding.**

NAME: **Marilyn Hayden**   Room number: **301-4**   Case number: Date: Signature

Person's Strengths: She can talk, at least part of message communicated, will keep trying—she knows she has trouble understanding, can walk

Behavior Management Plan

Behavior Trigger [cause of behavior]	Behavior	What works [Approaches]	Goals
PAIN degenerative changes spine arthritis knees with HX knee surgery & stiffness—lessened ROM	Resistant to care at times.	**CNAs** to approach gently and touch her prior to care—do not extend extremities beyond pain limit.	Staff will identify dementia pain signs -wringing hands. -fear of toilet Prevent pain during care.
	Difficulty sleeping every night.	**ALL** provide reassurance it is okay—touch her prior to care. Need preventive pain treatment & positioning at night to take weight off spine. Need elevated toilet seat. Whirlpool for days of increased soreness.	
HOSP SAYS AFRAID OF TOILET (using toilet hurts.)	Incontinent at times—using toilet hurts	Family to bring in arthritis friendly clothing.	Restore continence.
Loss of role of wife & mother & social contact as waitress.		**FAMILY** to make cassette tape of family voices & memory box with familiar objects Would Teddy bear or stuffed dog comfort her?	Provide her with a sense of home—familiarity.

NAME: **Marilyn Hayden**   Room number: **301-4**   Case number: Date: Signature

Person's Strengths: She can talk, at least part of message communicated, will keep trying—she knows she has trouble understanding, can walk

Behavior Management Plan

Behavior Trigger	Behavior	What works	Goals
[cause of behavior] Impaired vision Hard of hearing. Missed part of message. Poor short term memory. Lack of activities meaningful to her. **Complications: PAIN** Potential for depression due to: degenerative joint disease and diminished ability to dress, groom, bathe, eating, bed mobility & locomotion for distances..	Screaming "I don't know what to do" or "Why I'm here" 3 times a day TALKING to desk "What did I do to get here?" 3 times a day Daily pain which she communicates by being: Resistant to help and daily activities	[Approaches] **ALL** speak clearly and VERY LOUD but calm. Use 4 word sentences. REPEAT & REPEAT what you say. Offer 1 or 2 choices **Family** to bring in memory box **ACT** provide activities which do not depend on good hearing or vision. **ALL** touch her before moving her or providing care— anticipate her needs USE arthritis approach during care—gentle **SW** to evaluate for depression & get hearing evaluated & find her a friend. **Encourage her to wheel her WC down the hall to develop more strength.** **Pastoral minister visit.**	Resident will understand part of message on 3 out of 5 conversations daily. Make room "feel like home." She will have busy schedule during waking hours and something to do if she cannot sleep. Prevent pain and fear during care encounters. Staff will look for body language signals of pain and prevent pain. Res. will have exercise daily.

<u>NAME:</u> **Terry Jones**   <u>Room number: **223A**</u>   <u>Case number:</u>   <u>Date:</u>   <u>Signature</u>
Person's Strengths: Desire to communicate with others; Desire to understand what is happening; Desire to make choices.

Behavior Management Plan

Behavior Trigger [cause of behavior]	Behavior	What works	Goals
Pain (continued) Possible depression	**Verbally abusive** 1-3 days out of 7 **Physically abusive** 1-3 days out of 7	[Approaches] **NSG** to assess for pain when physically or verbally abusive. Caregivers will not grab her by her joints and will use arthritis friendly dressing, grooming and bathing techniques. **DR** to direct medication for pain prevention + identify & treat complicating problems. **Family** will bring in clothing with Velcro closures to allow her to participate in dressing. **DIET** to review nutritional status and recommend. **SW** will monitor signs and symptoms of improvement or worsening in mood state + behavior.	Verbal aggression will be reduced to weekly or less physical aggression will be reduced to weekly or less. She will not resist assistance in bathing, dressing and grooming activities in morning and evening daily. **Prevent pain** She will **participate in** dressing, bathing, grooming daily in morning and evening without pain. She will gain weight until within normal weight range for her. She will consume 75% or more of diet.

NAME: **Terry Jones**   Room number: **223A**   Case number: Date: Signature

Person's Strengths: Desire to communicate with others; Desire to understand what is happening; Desire to make choices.

Behavior Management Plan

Behavior Trigger [cause of behavior]	Behavior	What works [Approaches]	Goals
Assure him all his needs will be taken care of without pain.

Fear of the unknown he cannot remember
Being threatened by another confused man in the dining room 6-7.

Policemen by hx.
COMPLICATIONS:
HOH
IMPAIRED VISION

Altered taste due to dementia. | Verbal expressions of fear daily.

Pulled fire alarm 7/30 tried to pull fire alarm 1 year ago 7/20

Words of fear:
"They are trying to poison me." "Someone Is trying to kill me." | Assign the same caregivers daily. Follow a consistent routine daily. Give him a notebook where staff can write in what is done for him so he can see his needs are being met. **Assign** him to a small dining room away from the man who threatened him. **Anticipate cyclical pattern of pulling fire alarm.** Increase lighting but not glare in his room. Avoid noisy settings. **Staff** member to taste test food and show him it is okay. **Family** to bring in food. & seasoning. | **Reduce** verbal expression of fear to 3-4 times a week.

Staff will show him the notebook to reassure him.

He will not be in the same room with the man who scared him.

Maximize his ability to see and hear what is happening around him to lessen fear. |

NAME: **Joseph Marsac**   Room number: **221-1**   Case number: Date: Signature
Person's Strengths: He can talk, desire to do for himself, desire to make choices, supportive niece

Behavior Management Plan

Behavior Trigger	Behavior	What works	Goals
[cause of behavior] Arguing with him. harsh tone of voice. **MOD, PAIN DAILY** Not having a CNA or nurse he recognizes. He cannot remember. Desire to make choices. **+DO FOR HIMSELF**	If you argue with him, he swears and tries to bite + kick and hit. **Verbally abusive** 4-days a week. Refusing Care + medications 3 days out of 7.	[Approaches] **Do not argue**—talk about something else. Use a gentle tone of voice with kind words. Change the conversation to **what you want him to do**- Offer him more than one choice—he likes to choose what he will do. Give him something to do **Keep him busy.** **ACT** to offer him choices -would you rather read or pass out books to other people Help him find a friend **NSG-** Try pain meds. 20 minutes before AM care & before bedtime. **CNA** use arthritis friendly clothing— dress him gently avoiding hurting his back and limbs.	Reduce verbal outbursts to **3 times a week.** He will make choices about his life. Reduce his refusing care and meds. to 2 times a week or less. Prevent pain at least twice daily.

NAME: **Joseph Marsac**   Room number: **221-1**   Case number: Date: Signature

Person's Strengths: He can talk, desire to do for himself, desire to make choices, supportive niece

Behavior Management Plan

Behavior Trigger	Behavior	What works	Goals
[cause of behavior]	Doubling her fist.	[Approaches]	
Mary needs to have her "NO" accepted as a valid response.		STOP what you are doing and come back later to try again.	
	Sad worried daily.	DO NOT FORCE HER come back in 15 minutes and try again.	ALLOW HER TO MAKE CHOICES ABOUT CARE.
Arguing with her.	Hit, pinch caregivers.	Let her get up when she wants to.	
Expecting her to get up at the same time every day.	**Unhappy in morning 5x a week.**		She will not be unhappy in the morning.
Cluttered room or hallway, esp. if noisy.	**Wheels her wheelchair into people & walls.**	KEEP HER OUT OF HALLWAY WHEN NOISY & FULL OF PEOPLE. Keep her room clutter free.	
		Encourage her to wheel her wheelchair down the halls for exercise as long as she doesn't confront other residents.	She will not hit people or walls with her wheelchair
	Grunting.	Take her to quiet area—not her room, call her oompah (means grandma) touch her before moving her or providing care.	
Trying to ask for something OR upset about noise or clutter.	**Angry 5x a week.**	Speak to her in calm reassuring voice.	

NAME: **Mary Martin**   Room number: 303-1   Case number: Date: Signature

Person's Strengths: She wants to make her own choices, She wants to participate in her own care. She has strong family support.

Behavior Management Plan

Behavior Trigger [cause of behavior]	Behavior	What works [Approaches]	Goals
		Encourage her to attend busy hands activity in the morning and in the afternoon.	She will not hit people or walls with her wheel chair.
Polishing her nails. Putting her back to bed after meals.	Grunting, hitting clenched fist. **Grunting, hitting**.	Do not polish her nails. Do not put her back to bed after meals.	She will not hit. She will not be angry after meals.
Wants coffee or a drink.	**Tapping on tray**.	Give her coffee or a drink.	HONOR her requests when she makes them.
Not covering her legs with a lap quilt.	Clenched fist, grunting, hitting.	Cover her legs with a lap quilt when she is up in her wheelchair.	She will not be angry as evidenced by clenching her fist, grunting and hitting.

NAME: **Mary Martin**   Room number: 303-1   Case number: Date: Signature
Person's Strengths: She wants to make her own choices, She wants to participate in her own care. She has strong family support.

Deborah A. Bastedo

Behavior Management Plan

Behavior Trigger	Behavior	What works	Goals
[cause of behavior] PAIN Degenerative changes both shoulders and both humeri—prob. chronic per xray right hand. Osteopenia Tears rotator cuffs both shoulders per xray **Not on pain or anti-inflammatory medication** Misunderstands communication possibly due to aortic vascular calcification.	8/13 whining & wants to be in bed most of time daily. Crying. Verbally abusive 1-3 days out of 7. 6/4 mood changes cries for mother Resists care daily.	[Approaches] **NSG** to be very gentle with shoulders when assisting her with care **Family** to bring in clothing which buttons or snaps to avoid extension -soreness shoulders. Allow her to place her arms into sleeves and help in care. **DR & NSG** to monitor pain and determine effective preventive method-TRY routine pain RX 20 min. before AM care & 20 min. before bedtime.	Prevent and manage pain. Staff to recognize dementia expressions of pain: resisting care, crying, verbally abusive, not wanting to eat. Not to over extend shoulders as well as other joints. To give her feeling of control. **Reduce** verbal abuse to 1 time a week or less. Treat <u>pain</u> to determine if it is the <u>primary cause</u> of agitated behavior. Reduce resisting of care to 3 times a week or less.

<u>NAME</u>: **Karen Patillo**   <u>Room number</u>: **220A**   Case number: Date: Signature

Person's Strengths: She can talk, she can walk, family supportive

Behavior Management Plan

Behavior Trigger [cause of behavior]	Behavior	What works [Approaches]	Goals
Recently got worse—delirium? poss Urinary Tract Infection weight loss low albumin 5/3 poor teeth **Potential for depression** 6/18 wt loss 9/5 wt loss 3 lb	Socially inappropriate 1-3 days out of 7. Wanders 1-3 days out of 7. Eating less than 50% of meals.	**DR** evaluate and treat potential causes for enhanced confusion— **ALL** provide consistent routine daily. **Dentist** to treat teeth. **ACT** provide daily things for her to do—a quiet area where she can walk as much as she wants. **SW** visit & monitor for sadness. **Family** to do memory box & a tape with familiar voices on it. **Caregivers** to assist with eating if she does not eat 70& of meal or more without assist due to probably delirium status. **RD** to evaluate. **ALL** offer her water when with her	Heal other medical causes for confusion. Transform wandering into daily exercise program. Have surroundings feel like home. prevent further wt loss. Enhance nutritional status. Get her to drink fluids as she cannot remember to. Remove potential nutritional causes for delirium. Avoid pressure ulcers. **She** will eat 70% or more of meals.

NAME: **Karen Patillo**   Room number: **220A**   Case number: Date: Signature
Person's Strengths: She can talk, she can walk, family supportive

Deborah A. Bastedo

Behavior Management Plan

Behavior Trigger	Behavior	What works	Goals
[cause of behavior] **Giving her a shower.** Fear and anxiety over shower—hurts FEAR of potential pain PAIN-she hits the part that hurts. Soft tissue swelling ankle 7/31 E coli urine 9/16 pneumonia chronic COPD Hx breast concer poss. metastasis complicated by anemia—hgb 9.1 HX Cancer breast Possible constipation Low albumin	Combative during shower—even with Ativan prior Bangs chair into things. infection? Multiple skin tears. Resists care 4-6 days out of 7. Restlessness unable to sit still. **Physically abusive** 4-6 days out of 7. **Socially inappropriate** 1-3 days out of 7.	[Approaches] GIVING HER A BATH Be gentle in your approach do NOT tug or pull on arms & legs ***Pain management*** Very important as HX cause of anxiety—nursing to use dementia pain signs—restlessness, resisting care, hitting chair into things, combativeness. NSG to anticipate & prevent pain. TRY routine pain RX 20 min. before AM care before PM care **DIET** to provide fluids, and health shakes with meals.	**Mabel** will be clean and staff will be uninjured at least weekly. **ALL STAFF** to encourage pain relief positioning and calm, relaxing environment—praise calm responses. **DR** to resolve acute process and resolvable conditions. Reduce physical abuse to 2 times a week or less. Prevent pain during care. Get Mabel to allow care.

NAME: **Mabel Renshaw**   Room number: **205-2**   Case number: Date: 9-30   Signature
Person's Strengths: family supportive; desire to be free from pain; desire to make choices

98

Behavior Management Plan

Behavior Trigger [cause of behavior] **Depression** Possible acute process lungs 9/19 poss. Upper Respiratory Infection	Behavior Makes anxious statements; negative statements, repetitive statements "I don't know what I'm talking about. I don't know why I'm here" **Verbally abusive** 1-3 days out of 7.	What works [Approaches] **ALL** DO NOT ARGUE—this sets her off USE GENTLE HAPPY VOICE. MAKE EYE CONTACT. Encourage her to vent. Answer her factual questions. Provide her with a notebook where she can write down things she wishes to remember. Offer her choices. **SW** to provide visitation and reassurance her needs will be met. **Family** to visit & make a tape with family voices to make her room more like home—bring in familiar objects—pictures of family & tape player. **ACT** to play relaxing cassette tapes—meditation tapes. **DR** to treat infection.	Goals **Staff** will keep a picture of her on her door. **FAMILY** to give reassurance and provide needed home-like objects. **ALL** will encourage her to look things up in her notebook. **DIET** to monitor nutritional status and help prevent dehydration and pressure ulcers. **SW** to reassure **Verbal abuse will reduce to weekly or less.** **ACT** to provide alternatives to medication for anxiety relief. **Heal** infection to get down to primary dementia behavior.

NAME: **Mabel Renshaw**   Room number: **205-2**   Case number: Date: 9-30   Signature

Person's Strengths: family supportive; desire to be free from pain; desire to make choices

Behavior Management Plan

Behavior Trigger [cause of behavior]	Behavior	What works [Approaches]	Goals
PAIN Daily mild to moderate pain related to arthritis foot knees + related to curvature spine [unable to sleep at night]. **Complications:** Recurrent mouth lesions. Depression of long term illness. **Anxiety—fear** pain will not go away or that something done for her will hurt. Desire to be reassured everything is okay.	SAD pained expression, worried facial expressions up to 5 times a week. Crying, tearful up to 5 times a week. SAD, MOODS NOT EASILY ALTERED. Makes negative statements up to 5 times a week. Repeated health complaints up to 5 times a week.	Jobst pump anti-inflammatory pain medication elevating left leg after lunch. **CNA** will position her comfortably with pillows to take the pressure off her dorsal lumbar back at bedtime. DR suggested pillow under chest **ALL** validate concerns with health and respond with appropriate pain RX. Pain strategy—prevention. **NIECE** will make or buy a relaxation tape she can play & cassette player with ear phones so she can turn it up loud in order to try to use non-medical methods to relieve anxiety over chronic pain.	Negative statements, concerns with health, sad expressions and crying will decrease to 3 times a week **or less.** She will have medication & non medication relief for chronic pain available at all times. Staff will anticipate and prevent pain. Frances will voice pain free status daily. Frances will have non medicine pain relief available to her at all times.

<u>NAME</u>: **Frances Smith**   Room number: **123** Case number: Date: Signature

Person's Strengths: She can talk, establishes own goals, finds comfort in friends, clergy, family

Behavior Management Plan

Behavior Trigger [cause of behavior]	Behavior	What works [Approaches]	Goals
<u>Sadness over lost role in community and lost social status.</u> <u>Misses her accounting work at the Pontiac Motors.</u> **Hard of hearing uses hearing aid** **She had fight with her son and has not seen him since.** Fear that she will not be able to go back to apartment	Expresses anger— sadness empty feeling over: 1) lost role in community 2) Not feeling needed 3) strained relationship with family Tearfulness up to 5 times a week.	**Pastoral Minister** to visit to encourage her to express her spiritual beliefs and vent her fear. **SW** will encourage family to validate her feelings in order to help relieve anxiety & encourage peaceful relationship with son & make sure hearing aid has works & encourage friends from work to visit **ACT** will provide materials for in room activities when pain severe and encourage daily participation in regular activities esp. encourage empowerment activities + encourage Episcopalian church visitations. **FAMILY** will visit and bring her a tape with family voices to make her room feel more like home.	She will have a vent for her fear and anger concerns. She will put her concern over lost relationship with son to rest. She will have regular visits. She will have daily diversions which she enjoys. Her room will seem more like home to her.

NAME: **Frances Smith**   Room number: **123** Case number: Date: Signature
Person's Strengths: She can talk, establishes own goals, finds comfort in friends, clergy, family

Behavior Management Plan

Behavior Trigger [cause of behavior]	Behavior	What works [Approaches]	Goals
Pain due to degenerative changes in her bones according to x-rays. **Knees: hx total knee replacement, foot edema** **HX of FALL** due to high risk for another fall due to elevated blood pressure 6/16 & after and current use of Depakene 250mg twice a day, Risperdal 2 mg twice a day, Ativan 0.5mg twice a day. **Lasix 50 mg daily as needed.** (On admission she was only on Depakene.) <u>complicated by:</u> 8/8 ear infection 8/12 constipated.	8/13 Refusing to wear Mediboots. Resists care daily. Unable to communicate pain except by refusing care. dizziness 8/8 Loud restless. 8/8 Loud, verbal disputes. 8/14 Verbally abusive with roommate. **Needs more water** as indicated by constipation.	**NSG** to be very gentle with arms & legs when assisting her with care. **Family** to get clothing which buttons or snaps to avoid extension of arms and legs during dressing which causes pain. **DR & NSG** to monitor pain and determine effective treatment method-not on arthritis medicine or routine pain medicine. **DR and consultant DR** to decide if all 3 medications are necessary **ALL** offer her water when with her provide same routine daily. **DR** to evaluate and treat constipation & ear infection. **RD** to eval diet & amount of water **needed.**	Avoid pain during care. Treat pain routinely to determine if it is the primary cause of agitated behavior. **Focus on preventing pain.** **Reduce and or eliminate antipsychotic medications.** Evaluate her for use of antidepressant. She will receive a minimum 2500cc of water daily. Treat other medical causes for confusion Prevent further weight loss + enhance nutritional status.

<u>NAME: **Beth Stickney**</u>   <u>Room number: **207-3**</u>   <u>Case number:</u>   <u>Date:</u>   <u>Signature</u>

Person's Strengths: She can talk, she can express her needs, family supportive

Behavior Management Plan

Behavior Trigger [cause of behavior]	Behavior	What works [Approaches]	Goals
Depression complicated by: hydrocephalus	Picks fights with **roommate** "She sold my house" **daily**	**ACT** to provide daily things for her to do. Ask family for a tape with familiar voices on it & cassette player & memory box (**a box full of photos or familiar objects which she can handle and look at**). and pictures of family members.	Have surroundings feel like home. **Promote a sense of security.** Help her feel less isolated
Social isolation Lost roles mom—wife.		**SW** to place a picture of her on her door so she knows she lives there. **ALL** repeat back to her what she is saying and ask her what she, "things" we should do about her house being sold—let her vent. **SW** monitor for sadness & **HELP** her find a friend with common interests.	**Fights with roommate will end.** If trouble with roommate continues—find a different room or different roommate. Staff will encourage her to spend time with her new friend. She will have another interest. She will feel she belongs in her room and this is home.
Using regular toilet seat is too painful.	Urinates on floor in front of toilet & in chair	ELEVATED TOILET SEAT SO SHE WILL USE TOILET.	She will urinate in toilet.

NAME: **Beth Stickney**　　Room number: **207-3**　Case number:　　Date:　　Signature

Person's Strengths: She can talk, she can express her needs, family supportive

Behavior Management Plan

Behavior Trigger	Behavior	What works	Goals
[cause of behavior] Arguing with her. Harsh tone of voice. Desire to smoke. Desire to make choices. **Fear** her needs will not be met **especially smoking.** NO FAMILY so she looking for someone to care especially about her.	Gets on elevator without supervision hourly. If you argue with her she swears and tries to bite and hit. **Verbally abusive** 4-6 days a week. **Socially inappropriate** *daily* she spits on floor, furniture, urinates on chairs & plays in it. She says, "that lady doesn't love me" when people try to get her away from the elevator and argue with her. She will not change clothes esp. socks.	[Approaches] **Do not argue**—talk about something else—she cannot remember so reminding her not to get on the elevator is a waste of time—change the conversation to **what you want her to do.** Use a gentle tone of voice with kind words. Give her something to do **Keep her busy—she likes to help.** Offer her choices—would you rather read or pass out books to other people. Do NOT withhold smoking—*offer smoking as a reward* such as if she cooperates = "IF you change your socks, I'll take you down for a cigarette." Help her find a friend. Get a volunteer to visit her.	Reduce her attempts to get on the elevator to 3 every 8 hours. Reduce verbal outbursts to **3 times a week** or less. Reduce **daily** inappropriate behavior to 3-4 times a week. She will have someone to talk to so smoking will not be her only interest.

NAME: **Ethel Woods**   Room number: **238 B**   Case number: Date: Signature
Person's Strengths: She can talk, she can walk, desire to make choices, likes to smoke, likes to help, need for family

Behavior Management Plan

Behavior Trigger [cause of behavior]	Behavior	What works [Approaches]	Goals
Pain when clothing is changed.	**Verbally abusive** 4-6 days a week.	**DR-** Pain treatment before morning and bedtime care. **Caregiver** Use arthritis friendly clothing dress her gently. Avoiding hurting her back and limbs. Give her a notebook where staff write in what is done for her so she can see her needs are being met.	She will change her clothes **without hurting caregivers in the morning and at bedtime.**
She cannot remember.	**She says she does not get help and does not get what she needs.**		She will be able to see what is done for her even though she cannot remember what just happened. Assure her all her needs will be taken care of without pain.
She no longer understands it is not okay to spit on the floor. She does not understand what the "I have to pee" feeling "means."	**She spits on the floor several times daily.**	Provide her with an emesis basin and reward her when she uses it to spit in, such as take her for a cigarette.	
She needs something to do and touching familiar objects may make her feel more at home.	**She urinates on chairs daily and plays in it.**	Remind her and/or take her to the bathroom every 2-3 hours to use the toilet. Get her a raised toilet seat to see if she will use the toilet. Paint edge of seat a bright color so she can find it. **Prepare a box with objects she can manipulate, esp. pictures of her.**	She will use the emesis basin to spit in daily. She will not forget to use the toilet. She will use the toilet 2-4 times every 8 hours. She will remain clean & dry every 8 hours. She will have objects to manipulate.

NAME: **Ethel Woods**   Room number: **238 B**   Case number: Date: Signature

Person's Strengths: She can talk, she can walk, desire to make choices, likes to smoke, likes to help, need for family

Behavior Management Plan

Behavior Trigger [cause of behavior]	Behavior	What works [Approaches]	Goals

NAME:_____   Room number:_____   Case number: Date: Signature

Person's Strengths:

Bibliography:

Aronson, M.K. Understanding Alzheimer's Disease: What It Is, How to Cope With It, Future Directions. New York: Charles Scribner's Sons, 1988.

Babcock, Elise NeeDell. When Life Becomes Precious. New York: Bantam Books, 1997.

Boult, C. Comprehensive Geriatric Assessment. Whitehouse Station, NJ: The Merck Manual of Geriatrics. Retrieved 7-14-2001 from the World Wide Web.

http://www.merck.com/pubs/mm_geriatrics/sec1/ch4.htm

Comer, Ronald J. Abnormal Psychology. Second Edition, New York: W. H. Freeman and Company, 1995.

Dept. of Health & Human Services, HCFA; State Operations Manual April 1995.

Dipple, Raye Lynne, PhD and Hutton, J. Thomas, MD, PhD. Caring for the Alzheimer Patient. New York: Prometheus Books, 1996.

Doka, Kenneth J. with Davison, Joyce [editors]. Living with Grief When Illness Is Prolonged. Bristol, PA: Taylor & Francis, 1997.

Frank, J. D. & Frank, J. B. Persuasion and Healing, A Comparative Study of Psychotherapy (3rd ed.) Baltimore: The John Hopkins University Press. 1991.

Goldberg, Irene and Goldberg, Herbert, Family Therapy: An Overview. California: Brooks/Cole Publishing Company, 1996.

Kalb, C. Coping With Darkness, Revolutionary New Approaches in Providing Care and Helping People with Alzheimer's Stay Active and Feel Productive. Newsweek, CXXXV (no.5), 52-55. 2000, 1-31.

Koenig, Harold. Aging, Spirituality, and Religion: A Handbook. "Religion and Health in Later Life".

Kouri, Mary K., PhD. Keys To Survival For Caregivers. New York: Barron's Educational Series, Inc., 1992.

Lemonick, M. D. & Mankato, A. P. THE NUN STUDY, How One Scientist and 678 Sisters are Helping Unlock the Secrets of ALZHEIMER'S. Time Magazine. 157 (19), 54-64.

Reichlin, R. E. Integrated Group Approaches with the Early Stage Alzheimer's Patient and Family. In M. Duffy, PhD (Ed.) Handbook of Counseling and Psychotherapy with Older Adults (1st ed., pp. 166-181). New York: John Wiley & Sons, Inc., 1999.

Rose, Larry. Show Me The Way To Go Home. Forest Knolls, California: Elder Books, 1996.

Voss-Morice, Sidney, RN, MSN. GERIATRIC NURSING. Aurora, Colorado: Skidmore-Roth Publishing, Inc., 1996.

Deborah A. Bastedo

REALLY GREAT BOOKS:

<u>**Show Me The Way To Go Home**</u>, by Larry Rose. Forest Knolls, California: Elder Books, 1996.

Larry Rose has a genius IQ and is a member of Mensa (a group which requires members to have high Intelligence Quotients.) In this book, written by Mr. Rose his editor and his wife, he chronicles his Alzheimer disease and what it feels like to have it. Very readable. I read it in a single evening. I could not put it down.

<u>**Understanding Difficult Behaviors**</u>, by Ann Robinson, Laurie White and Beth Spencer. This book is like a dictionary of behavior problems with possible solutions. It is the result of research as well as years of working with demented people. An excellent resource. This book can be obtained from **Eastern Michigan University** Alzheimer's Education Program by calling: 734-487-2335 or FAX 734-487-0298 or write:

EMU Alzheimer's Education Program
P. O. Box 981337
Ypsilanti, MI 48198-1337   **Visa and Mastercard accepted.**

<u>**The Validation Breakthrough**</u> by Naomi Feil

Activity Directors indicate this book to be quite useful. It is about the way a person talks to a confused person. It can be ordered through Briggs Corporation, call 1-800-247-2343. If you hear a message which says you cannot use this number from your area code, it means they are not open on the day you called or not open yet for that day.

<u>**Alzheimer's Disease, Activity-Focused Care**</u> by Carly R. Hellen

Carly is an Occupational Therapist and explores innovative ideas for promoting life's meaning and personhood, valuing the victim of this disease as well as support group ideas. She encourages using ideas for exercise and mobility to promote self-esteem. Available through Butterworth Heinmann Press at webside http://www.bh.com or 225 Wildwood Avenue; Woburn, MA 01801-2041 Phone: 718-904-2500 Fax: 718-904-2620.

<u>**The Complete Guide to Alzheimer's-Proofing Your Home**</u> By Mark L. Warner Mr. Warner is an architect and gerontologist. He creates safer homes for senior citizens and this book contains many useful suggestions for ways you can make your homes safer and life easier when caring for a person with dementia. For example, he suggests placing a magazine picture of silverware on your silverware drawer so that the demented family member can find the silverware. This is a publication of Purdue University Press, West Lafayette, Indiana.

<u>**A Life Worth Living. Practical Strategies for Reducing Depression in Older Adults**</u> by Pearl Mosher-Ashley & Phyllis Barrett $29.95 Wellness Productions 1-800-501-8120.

<u>**More Than Movement for Fit to Frail Older Adults.**</u> by Pauline Postiloff Fisher. $ 22.95 Wellness Productions. 1-800-501-8120

<u>**Stretch & Strengthen for Rehabilitation and Development.**</u> by Bob Anderson & Donald Bornell, Stretching, Inc. 1-800-333-1307 website and online store: www.stretching.com

Stretching: the Video by Bob Anderson Stretching, Inc. 1-800-333-1307 website and online store: www.stretching.com

Tai Chi for Seniors with Master Xue Dejun video $20. Harmony Catalogue 1-800-869-3446 also available at: www.gaiam.com

Make A Difference...A Practical Approach to Dementia Care by Deborah Bastedo and Angela Willis This book is written with love from the daughters of dementia victims. It contains ideas for problem solving, considerations for assessment and resources for families and victims. It is available from Bastedo, MRS, Inc (248) 682-7480; 1069 Pelham Blvd.; Waterford, MI 48328-4262 **Visa and Mastercard accepted**

The Relaxation Response. by Herbert Benson, M.D. How to use a simple meditative technique to cope with fatigue, anxiety and stress.

Free Booklets:

The Agency for Health Care Policy and Research, an agency of the U. S. Department of Health and Human Services, supported the development of guidelines for people and caregivers relating to a specific problem. These guidelines and others are available to public by calling: **800-358-9295** or write to:

Agency for Health Care Policy and Research
Publications Clearinghouse
P. O. Box 8547
Silver Spring, MD 20907

Depression Is a Treatable Illness: Patient Guide discusses major depressive disorder, which usually can be treated successfully with the help of a health professional. (AHCPR Publication No. 93-0053)

Recovering After a Stroke: Patient and Family Guide tells how to help a person who has had a stroke achieve the best possible recovery. (AHCPR Publication No. 93-0664)

Understanding Urinary Incontinence in Adults: Patient Guide describes why people lose urine when they don't want to and what can be done about it. (AHCPR Publication No. 96-0684)

Preventing Pressure Ulcers: Patient Guide discusses symptoms and causes of bed sores and ways to prevent them. (AHCPR Publication No. 92-0048)

Treating Pressure Sores: *Consumer Guide* describes basic steps of care for bed sores. (AHCPR Publication No. 95-0654)

Resources for Patients and Families:

Administration on Aging
330 Independence Avenue, SW
Washington DC 20201
(202) 619-1006
Internet: http://www.aoa.dhhs.gov

Alzheimer's Association
919 North Michigan Avenue
Suite 100
Chicago, IL 60611-1676
(312) 335-8700
800-272-3900
Internet: http://www.alz.org

Alzheimer's Disease Education and Referral (ADEAR) Center:
P. O. Box 8250
Silver Spring, MD 20907-8250
800-438-4380
Internet: adear@alzheimers.org

American Association of Retired Persons (AARP)
Washington DC
(202) 424-2277
800-424-3410

Children of Aging Parents
Levittown, PA
(215) 945-6900

The Corporation for National Service
Office of Public Liaison
1201 New York Avenue, NW
Washington, DC 20525
(202) 606-5000

Eldercare Locator
Washington DC
800-677-1116

Insurance Consumer Helpline
Washington, DC
800-942-4242

Medicare Hotline
Baltimore, MD
800-638-6833

National Association For Continence (formerly Help for Incontinent People) Spartinburg, SC
(800) 252-3337
800-BLADDER

National Hospice Organization
Arlington, VA
(703) 243-5900
800-658-8898

"Spiritual Well-Being is the affirmation of life in a relationship with God, self, community and environment that nutures and celebrates wholeness."
Copyright 1975 NICA

National Interfaith Coalition on Aging, Inc. (NICA)
298 S. Hull St.
P. O. Box 1924
Athens, GA 30603

National Parkinson's Foundation
East Coast: Miami, FL
800-327-4545
West Coast: Encino, CA
800-522-8855

National Stroke Association
Englewood, CO
(303) 771-1700
800-STROKES

Reach Study Webside
http://www.edu.reach/

Social Security Information
800-772-1213
(open 7 am - 7 pm in all time zones)

U. S. Department of Veterans Affairs
Regional Office, Veterans Assistance
Washington, DC
(202) 418-4343
800-827-1000

RESOURCES FOR ASSISTIVE DEVICES

PHONES:

Intenna Cordless Phone	Cobra: 800-262-7222
Portable Telephone Amplifier	AT & T phone Center
Remote Access Speaker Phone	Maxi-Aids: 800-522-6294
Voice Print Phone	Maxi-Aids: 800-522-6294

Back Talk	HARC Mercantile, Ltd.: 800-445-9968
	available through LS & S Group, Inc.
	800-468-4789

Picture Phone   **Can-Do Products: 800-537-2118**

Closed Circuit Television Systems CTECH:	800-421-7323 (Optelec 20/20)
Large Print Keytop Labels	Hoolean Corporation 800-937-1337
Anti-Glare Screen Device VDT Visor	AliMed Inc.: 800-937-1337
Character Enlargement System for Computer Vista	Telesensory Corp.:
	800-227-8418

DECtalk Express External Synthesizer	EVAS: 800-872-3827
Perfect Reader	Maxi-Aids: 800-522-6294
Listenaider Hearing Assistive Device	**Maxi-Aids:** **800-522-6294**
Sonic Alert System	Maxi-Aids: 800-522-6294

Quiet Wake	National Flashing Systems: 301-589-6671
Range Queen	Pyro-Control Inc.: 817-335-5981
Guardian Net IV	Guardian Electronics, Ltd.: 414-241-4850
Intercom/Electric Door Release	Nutone: 800-543-8687

Automatic Medication Dispenser   CompuMed: 800-722-4417

X-10 Powerhouse	X-10 (USA) Inc.800-526-0027
Allegro Remote Control	Bruce Health & Med. Supplies:
	800-225-8446
Guardian Tub Lift	Guardian 800-255-5022
Transfer handle	Mobility Transfer Systems, Inc.
	800-854-4687
Dressing/bathing/grooming aids	Sammons Catalogue:
	800-323-5547
Meal Preparations Aids	Sammons Catalogue: 800-323-5547
Off-Set Door Hinge	Sammons Catalogue: 800-323-5547

Love Lift   **Love Lift: 800-456-8826**
Floor Model Patient Lift   Barrier-free Lifts, Inc. 800-582-8732

Automatic Card Shuffler	Adaptability: 800-266-8856
Cardholder	The Lighthouse, Inc.: 800-829-0500
Cone checkers	Adaptability: 800-266-8856
Knitting Aid	Access to Recreation: 800-634-4351
Scald Safe	**Resources Conservation: 800-243-2862**

About the Author

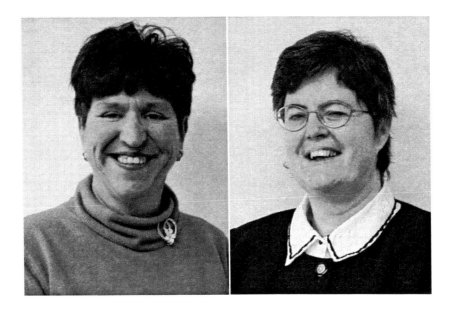

Angela Willis is a registered nurse, a licensed nursing home administrator with a master's degree in skilled nursing and is currently completing her doctorate. Her passion for the elderly led to her interest in victims of dementia. She has an instinct for finding ways to assist dementia victims have a better quality of life. She took care of her mother who was a victim of Alzheimer's disease, while at the same time raising a family. Her objective is to serve as ambassador for victims of dementia and their families and help others to see them with love as she does.

A passion for people led Deborah Bastedo to earn a master's degree in counseling as well as earn her Mental Health Specialty. She is a licensed and Nationally Certified Counselor. Dementia became her focus because of her father's diagnosis of Alzheimer's disease fifteen years ago. Her experience includes being called in to assist a nursing home find alternatives to anti-psychotic medication for more than eighty patients. Her motivation is to assist caregivers in using dementia-friendly approaches for environmental and behavioral management of dementia victims. She has three grown children, but, she says, "My husband still needs a little tweaking."